PASTEST
Dedicated to your success

© 2004 PASTEST Ltd
Egerton Court
Parkgate Estate
Knutsford
Cheshire
WA16 8DX

Telephone: 01565 752000

First published 2004

ISBN: 1 904627 11 0

A catalogue record for this book is available from the British Library.

The information contained within this book was obtained by the authors from reliable sources. However, while every effort has been made to ensure its accuracy, no responsibility for loss, damage or injury occasioned to any person acting or refraining from action as a result of information contained herein can be accepted by the publishers or authors.

PasTest Revision Books and Intensive Courses
PasTest has been established in the field of postgraduate medical education since 1972, providing revision books and intensive study courses for doctors preparing for their professional examinations.

Books and courses are available for the following specialties:
MRCGP, MRCP Parts 1 and 2, MRCPCH Parts 1 and 2, MRCPsych, MRCS, MRCOG Parts 1 and 2, DRCOG, FRCA, PLAB Parts 1 and 2.

For further details contact:
PasTest, Knutsford, Cheshire WA16 7BR
Tel: 01565 752000   Fax: 01565 650264
www.pastest.co.uk   enquiries@pastest.co.uk

Text prepared by Carnegie Book Production, Lancaster
Printed and bound in Europe by The Alden Group

Contents

OSCE Stations

Answers with explanations and comments

Contributors

Adam Feather MB MRCP
Senior Lecturer in Medical Education
St Bartholomew's and The Royal London Hospital Medical School
Consultant Physician
Newham Healthcare Trust
London

John S P Lumley MS FRCS
Professor of Vascular Surgery
University of London
Honorary Consultant Surgeon
Great Ormond Street Children's Hospital
Medical College and Hospital of St Bartholomew, London
Member of Council, Royal College of Surgeons of England
Past World President, International College of Surgeons

Ramanathan Visvanathan BM BCh FRCS ILTM
Consultant Surgeon
Bronglais General Hospital
Aberystwyth
SY23 1ER
And Breast Test Wales, Swansea
Honorary Lecturer, University of Wales College of Medicine
Surgical Tutor, Royal College of Surgeons of England

Jonathan Round BA MBBS MRCP
Senior Lecturer in Child Health
Graduate Entry Program
St George's Hospital Medical School
Cranmer Terrace
Tooting
London
SW17 0RE

Kevin Hayes
Lecturer in Medical Education and Obstetrics and Gynaecology
St George's Hospital Medical School
Cranmer Terrace
Tooting
London
SW17 0RE

Angela Hall BSc Postgrad DipSoc
Senior Lecturer in Clinical Communications
Department of Medical Health Care Education
St George's Hospital Medical School
Cranmer Terrace
Tooting
London
SW17 0RE

Acknowledgements

These volumes would not have reached their present high standards without the excellent contribution made by Angela Hall, Senior Lecturer in Communication Skills at St George's Hospital Medical School. Her expert advice on the process elements of all the communication skills stations have improved the quality and have helped to produce stations which truly reflect those used at the majority of UK medical schools at final MBBS. Whilst the style of OSCE checklists will no doubt evolve over the next few years the elements she has included will not. We are very grateful to her for her expert contribution.

We are grateful to the excellent contribution made to this volume by Kevin Hayes, MRCOG. His expertise in Obstetrics and Gynaecology and the assessment of final year medical students have led to a greatly improved chapter on Obstetrics and Gynaecology.

Preface

Followers of recent literature on the assessment of undergraduate medical training could be excused for thinking that traditional methods were incomplete, if not arbitrary, and that potentially harmful doctors were being let loose on an unsuspecting public. This opinion is based on the immeasurable nature of 'gut feeling' in the marking of an essay and assessing clinical competence. The application of objective measurement in qualifying examinations does add credibility to their outcome.

Every examination must be fair and favour the well-prepared, ie valid and reliable. We have discussed the relative merits of essays, SAQs and MCQs elsewhere, this book, (and its companion volumes), is directed at the use of OSCEs in medicine. It provides a means of assessing practical procedures and communication skills, as well as knowledge and attitudes in most aspects of training.

The book is aimed at students preparing for their exit examination and will provide experience in this now widely-used examination technique. The book will also help those setting OSCE questions, providing a template onto which they can develop their own themes. OSCEs can assess history, examination, investigation and treatment of disease, together with practical techniques. OSCE stations can also obtain information on attitudes, interpersonal skills and ethical opinions. Some of these stations require the use of standard patients, manikin and videos. Although these media are not all reproduceable in a text book, advice is given on the way to deal with the likely questions, techniques and style of stations that may be encountered. It indicates what the examiner is looking for and how marks are being allocated for the approach to a patient and empathy with their problem. A correct diagnosis is not necessarily the key to obtaining a satisfactory mark: always remember to read the instructions very carefully.

The book follows a systems approach and each chapter includes questions from each type of OSCE station. Space is left for the student to respond to each question. Answers and additional advice are given in a separate section, allowing the students to assess their performance and identify areas needing further attention. In keeping with other books in the series, a revision checklist is given, and mock examinations are laid out: these latter can be undertaken within a prescribed time schedule and used for self-assessment.

Preface to the Second Edition

A chapter of paediatric stations and an extended chapter in obstetrics and gynaecology have been added in these new editions, increasing the series to three volumes. At the request of students, checklists have been included at the beginning of each chapter and there have been minor stylistic changes.

The marking system in most undergraduate examinations is item-based, although many schools are moving towards the standard postgraduate domain-based assessment, such as of generic skills and examining a region of the body; the text reflects these changing practices.

An interesting and desirable development has been the move back towards structured short cases, with emphasis on diagnostic skills, rather than process. The text also reflects these changes, as seen from the additional examiner's questions in many stations.

Units have not been included in the questions but tables of normal values are included at the beginning of each volume.

Introduction

Traditional methods of assessing knowledge and clinical skills have been based on the essay and MCQ, for written tests, and the long cases, short cases and the viva for practical aspects. These forms of assessment have been extensively challenged as to their ability to test and rank students. The essay has come under the greatest criticism but the long and short cases have also been questioned as to their objectivity and reliability. Marking a viva can be very subjective and it provides a very patchy assessment of the curriculum.

Objective structured clinical examinations (OSCEs) have been designed to provide a broader coverage of knowledge and skills in a quantifiable, valid and reliable form. They aim to assess interpretive skills, as well as factual recall; they include task-orientated items and they can examine a candidate's powers of decision making and their behavioural attitude in simulated professional practice. The overall effect is to provide a more valid assessment of candidates for their subsequent clinical practice.

The OSCE comprises a number of stations, through which a group of students rotate. The number of students in the examination usually matches the number of stations, so that by the end of the examination, each student has visited every station. There may be more stations than candidates without disturbing the organisation of the examination. Usually the time allowed for each station is the same throughout but it can be increased by inserting rest or preparatory stations before a longer question. Rest stations may also be used to provide natural breaks and to increase the number of candidates being examined at any one time.

The time at a station is usually at least three minutes, five minutes being common; 24 stations are available for a two hour examination. For an examination to be statistically reliable there must be a minimum of 17–20 stations. Formative assessments may use a few selected stations (eg 5–10). The design of OSCE questions is usually only limited by the ingenuity of the examiners. However, questions should examine a specific part of the curriculum, rather than just an ability to respond to the style of the examination. Students should be exposed to all proposed designs of question format before the final examination.

Each station of an OSCE should assess a discrete skill. This may be a basic test of practical ability or knowledge, or involve a higher level of thinking. It is wise to have a range of difficulty to help discriminate within a group. A number of questions are included to assess core knowledge: all students are expected to pass these stations. The clinical skills of diagnosis and treatment can be divided up into:

- taking a history
- performing an examination
- requesting appropriate investigations
- making the diagnosis
- assessing the severity of the disease
- prescribing treatment.

The latter should incorporate all aspects of care, including medicine, surgery, nursing and other medical and paramedical disciplines.

The history may be taken from a standardised patient (SP), or presented as a written scenario or a video. SPs may be simulated or actual patients. In the former, a well individual is trained to simulate a patient's illness in a standard way, portraying a patient's problems. Some training is usually required for actual patients, to ensure that the main points are brought out on request and that a history can be covered fully within the time allowed for that station. Simulated patients are usually actors, although sometimes students may act as SPs. In so doing students learn the evaluation process by direct observation and listening to presentations. These stations are usually manned by an examiner who is watching and listening, not only to the style of questioning, but also to student/patient interrelationships, their conversational skills, interpersonal skills, behaviour, attitude and psychomotor assessment. SPs are often asked to give their marks on the student encounter. Written scenarios can form the basis of subsequent questions, along the line of structured answer questions. They can test factual knowledge, understanding and cognitive skills but assess clinical competencies to a variable extent. Well-trained actors can become skilled historians and very persuasive patients, such as when replicating a psychiatric disturbance, although the latter are often more effectively covered with video sequences.

Examination of a patient in a manned station is a very valuable form of assessment. However, it also presents a great problem to the examiner, since very few conditions can be repeatedly examined for two hours at a time, and the number of conditions that can be easily replicated is limited, particularly if there are a number of groups of students being examined simultaneously or consecutively. Fit models can be used for the demonstration of a normal examination and normal anatomy or, alternatively, manikins can be available to assess specific examination techniques such as rectal and vaginal assessment.

A text book has difficulty in reproducing a history and examination, in view of their practical nature and the requirement of simulated patients, videos and models. This book does, however, consider the likely SPs, historical scenarios and types of models and manikins, and the examination techniques that are encountered in OSCEs. Investigations and their interpretation can easily be presented in OSCE form, and candidates can expect charts, and lists of haematological and biochemical results, together with all forms of radiological investigations, with a request to interpret data and radiological abnormalities.

OSCE stations are suitable for most aspects of treatment and prognosis. It is essential to remember that treatment of a 'medical' illness should not be limited to drugs or that of a 'surgical' illness to surgery alone. They should include all forms of available and desirable intervention. This avoids the 'pigeon-holing' of disease entities into conventional specialities which is deprecated in current clinical teaching. Counselling skills and the assessment of ethical factors in clinical practice are readily tested in an OSCE setting as SPs can provide both the background and the patient's attitude to an illness. The practical application of clinical skills and procedures are also readily assessed, usually with the aid of a manikin which allows such procedures as venous catheterization, cardiopulmonary resuscitation, securing and maintaining an air-way, wound debridement and suturing.

Desirable Features of OSCEs

OSCEs bring a new dimension to the assessment of medical training. Of particular value is their ability to examine practical and other skills in a unified, measurable and reproducible fashion. This is in keeping with current trends towards performance based assessment throughout health care. OSCEs provide for an effective use of the examination time, examiners' time and commitment. They are effective in assessing knowledge and practical skills and ensure that each student is presented with the same material, thus providing a uniform evaluation with consistent marking of all those involved.

The validity of the response to each question is primarily related to the student's ability: in well constructed questions, very little variation is dependent on the examiner's responses in manned stations. The reliability of OSCEs in differentiating good from bad students and the inter-rater reliability of examiners is good, and becomes increasingly certain as the number of stations devoted to each component part is increased. Both construct and content validity have been well established.

Well constructed questions are durable and can stand up to repeated use without weakening their value. Like many forms of assessment, effective questions represent the core curriculum material, and once a suitable bank size has been achieved, security of the questions is unnecessary as knowledge of the answers represents a passable understanding of the curriculum. Experiments on presenting a single station at a time to groups of students have not reduced their value in differentiating clinical performance. Assessment can be by the students themselves or by peer review. This modification substantially reduces the necessary space and organisation for an OSCE.

OSCEs can be a useful teaching modality. With the reduced stay of patients in hospitals and increased community-based education, medical schools often have to extend their teaching practice onto a number of sites. All these factors increase the need for uniformity of teaching methods as well as assessment. This can be effectively achieved with the use of OSCEs, and the reduced number of available patients can be addressed by the use of standard patients with good effect. One well-proven example of the use of simulated patients has been in the training and assessment of trauma, linked to the Advanced Trauma Life Support and related programmes. The use of students as SPs has proved an important and enjoyable learning experience, as well as, in some cases, providing financial rewards.

- Construct validity is the ability of the OSCE to differentiate students' ability, or to follow a student's progress before and after a course of instruction.
- Content (criterion-based) validity assesses the value of the station in reaching its specified objective. In all these measures OSCEs have proved effective in student assessment and are accepted by staff and students as a fair and desirable form of assessment.

Assessment is a powerful learning tool and should be used as part of the teaching and learning processes but it must be accompanied by adequate feedback in order to benefit individual students. This process should also be used in auditing teaching methods and to stimulate any necessary changes. It is feasible to set up OSCEs in any medical school, provided appropriate staff time is allowed for their introduction. Some schools involve students in the design and development of OSCEs and it can increase their awareness of this form of assessment. The formulation of OSCEs should be closely linked with curriculum development and keyed into the curriculum objectives.

When using OSCEs to evaluate teaching methods, two types of error should be considered.

- Type I errors are those of fact, implying a deficiency of teaching and/or learning, reflecting omissions and ineffective or absent experience.
- Type II errors are defects of understanding, where a student fails to recognise or interpret a clinical situation. This reflects poor concept attainment and an inability to discriminate.

Locating these errors points to the direction that future teaching should follow.

Disadvantages of OSCEs

As discussed in the previous section, the value of OSCEs in training and assessment has been demonstrated in many fields and many such assessment packages are available. However, medical schools should not become involved in this form of assessment without allowing adequate staff time for their development and OSCEs should not become the only form of assessment.

The preparation of OSCEs requires a good deal of thought and time. The whole staff should be aware of, and preferably involved in, their development and students should have experience prior to any examination so that they can be comfortable with this form of assessment. An OSCE requires a great deal of organisation in collecting material, appropriate patients, laying out stations and making sure staff are available for manned areas. Setting up the examination can be costly on administration and on medical staff and patients, and includes the hidden costs of Faculty time in the development of the exercise.

Analysis of the data and ensuring the validity of the examination requires painstaking activity. The weighting of key questions on essential knowledge has to be resolved before any feedback to staff or students. Standard setting should be based on expected knowledge and the skills required and this relies as much on that much-criticized 'gut feeling' as it does on statistical formulae. Standardised patients, both actual and simulated have to be found and trained and an adequate pool must be available to cover expected needs. When introducing OSCEs, a school has to decide whether it is as an additional assessment or whether it should replace a previous part of the examination. If the latter, it is essential that other important areas are not diluted in the process. OSCEs are not ideal in assessing interpersonal skills: video clips or trained patients can be rather artificial in this respect. For patient examination, OSCEs do not provide a comprehensive evaluation of all aspects of a learning and educational programme and therefore should be part of a multi-component assessment in the final examination, forming a useful means of determining practical skills over a wide area.

In spite of their potential limitations, OSCEs do provide a valuable addition to the clinical exit examination and students and staff should become well acquainted with their format and appreciate their discriminatory properties.

How to Use this Book

This book contains a series of OSCE questions. The chapters are arranged by organ system, and every chapter follows the same organisation of questions, i.e. history, examination, investigation, treatment, practical techniques and other issues. The second half of the book provides the answers, together with teaching notes and a marking scheme. There is no index but the contents list will direct you to the appropriate organ system.

In the history and counselling stations, you are advised to work with one to two colleagues to act as 'patient' and 'examiner'. The Introduction provides the background required to direct your enquiry or your counselling. Take a history from the 'patient', who will answer your questions using the history provided. The 'examiner' will mark your answers, using the scoring system outlines below, and ensure that the station is concluded in the allotted time.

The clinical examination stations include clinical photographs and test clinical skills which can be practised on appropriate patients on the ward. As the practical skills of examination cannot be assessed by a text book, a check list is included, indicating what the examiner is looking for in your examination of each system. The radiographic questions may be self-assessed by turning to the answer section.

Stations with radiographs or photographs may also carry statements requiring a 'true' or 'false' response. This adds variety to the station format and requires you to assess the answers given with respect to the radiograph or photograph. Similarly, stations with tables depicting clinical scenarios or treatment regimes test your knowledge in rearranging the latter to fit the disease.

At the back of the book there is a section that explains the marking schedule used for the stations, and a mock exam that contains five 19-station OSCE circuits: these provide typical examination scenarios.

By working through each organ system, as denoted by the chapters, you will cover most of the OSCE station scenarios and variations that you can expect to encounter in the undergraduate course.

Scoring your performance

We have chosen not to weight individual questions or items. Good is allocated 3 marks and adequate 2. In the poor/not done column the assessor can differentiate between a reasonable but inadequate mark and poor or not done. This differentiation can direct future study requirements. Each station is allocated the same mark, item scores are added in three column answers. Two of three correct responses or a mean score of 2 is a pass. A 60% correct response rate is required in two column answers. In the mock examinations two-thirds of stations should be passed to pass the examination.

Glossary

A-level	Advanced Level General Certificate of Education – School leaving Examination
ABGs	Arterial blood gases
AC	Abdominal circumference
ACE inhibitors	Angiotensin converting enzyme
ACTH	Adrenocorticotrophic hormone
Ach	Acetylcholine
ACS	Acute coronary syndrome
ADH	Anti-diuretic hormone
ADL	Activity of daily living
AF	Atrial fibrilation
AFP	Alpha-fetoprotein
aGBM	Anti-glomerular basement membrane
AGT	Angiotensin
AIDS	Acquired immune deficiency syndrome
AKA	Also known as
Alb	Albumin
Alk phos	Alkaline phosphatase
ALT	Alanine amino-transferase
AMA	Antimitochondrial antibody
ANCA	Anti neutrophil cytoplasmic antibody
Anti dsDNA	Double stranded deoxyribonucleic acid
Anti-Jo	Specific antigen
Anti-La	Specific antigen
Anti-RNP	Ribonucleic protein
Anti-Ro	Specific antigen
Anti-SCL70	Specific antigen
AP	Antero-posterior
APC gene	Adenomatosis polyposis coli
APTT	Activated partial thromboplastin time
ARDS	Adult respiratory distress syndrome
ARM	Artificial rupture of membranes
AS	Aortic stenosis
ASH	Action on smoking and health
ASMA	anti- smooth muscle antibody
ASO(T)	Anti streptolysin-O-titre
AST	Aspartate amino-transferase
ATLS	Advanced trauma life support
AV	Arterio-venous

AV	Atrio-ventricular
aVF	Augmented voltage lead left lower leg
aVL	Augmented voltage lead left arm
aVR	Augmented voltage lead right arm
AVSD	Atrioventricular septal defect
AXR	Abdominal X-ray
AZT	Azidothymidine (Generic Name: Zidovudine)
BAL	Broncho-alveolar lavage
BBB	Bundle branch block
BCC	Basal cell carcinoma
BCG	Bacille Calmette-Guerin
b.d.	Bis die (twice daily)
BE	Base excess
BHL	Bilateral hilar lymphadenopathy
BMA	British Medical Association
BM stix	Blood monitoring
BM	Bone marrow
BMI	Body mass index
BMR	Basal metabolic rate
BP	Blood pressure
Bpm	Beats per minute
BRCA	Breast cancer susceptibility genes
C	Cervical
Ca	Cancer
CA	Cyclic AMP
Ca2+	Calcium
CAGE questionnaire	Cut down Annoyed Guilty Eye-opener
CANCA	Anti-neutrophil cytoplasmic antibody
CAPD	Chronic ambulatory peritoneal dialysis
CCa^{2+}	Corrected calcium
CD4	A surface antigen principally found on helper-inducer T-lymphocyte
CEA	Carcinoembryonic antigen
CEMD	Confidential Enquiry into Maternal Health
CESDI	Confidential Enquiry into Stillbirths and Deaths in Infancy
CF	Cystic fibrosis
CIN I II III	Cervical intraepithelial neoplasia
CK	Creatinine phosphokinase
Cl	Chloride
CLL	Chronic lymphocytic leukaemia
Cm	Centimetre
CML	Chronic myeloid leukaemia

CMV	Cytomegalovirus
CNS	Central nervous system
CO2	Carbon dioxide
COCP	Combined oral contraceptive pill
COMT	Catechol O-methyl transferase
CPN	Community psychiatric nurse
CPR	Cardio pulmonary resuscitation
Cr	Creatinine
CREST	Crest syndrome – calcinosis; Raynaud's; oesophageal dysmotility; sclerodactyly; telangiectasia
CS	Caesarean section
CSF	Cerebro-spinal fluid
CSU	Catheter specimen of urine
CT	Computerised tomography
CTG	Cardiotocography
CVA	Cerebro-vascular accident
CVP	Central venous pressure
CVS	Chorionic villi sampling
CWD	Consistent with dates
CXR	Chest radiograph
DDAVP	Desmopressin, synthetic vasopressin
DIC	Disseminated intravascular coagulopathy
DIP joints	Distal inter-phalangeal joints
DKA	Diabetic keto-acidosis
dl	Decilitres
DM	Diabetes mellitus
DMSA	Dimercaptosuccinic acid
DNA	Deoxyribonucleic acid
DTP	Diphtheria-tetanus pertussis (vaccine)
DU	Duodenal ulcer
DVT	Deep vein thrombosis
DVLA	Driving vehicle licensing authority
ECG	Electrocardiogram
EEG	Electroencephalogram
EMQ	Extended matching question
ENT	Ear, nose and throat
ERCP	Endoscopic retrograde cholangiopancreatography
ESR	Erythrocyte sedimentation rate
ETEC	Enterotoxigenic Escherichia coli
EUA	Examination under anaestesia
FBC	Full blood count
FEV1	Forced expiratory volume in one second

FFP	Fresh frozen plasma
FH	Family history
5-FU	5-Fluoro-uracil
5HT	5-hydroxy-tryptamine
fl	Femtolitres
F:M	Female:male (ratio)
FNA	Fine needle aspirate
FPC	Family planning clinic
FSH	Follicular stimulating hormone
fT4	Free thyroxine
FVC	Forced vital capacity
GABA	Gamma- amino butyric acid
GCS	Glasgow coma score
GCSE	General Certificate of Secondary Education
GCSF	Granulocyte colony stimulating factor
GDM	Gestational diabetes mellitus
GI	Gastrointestinal
GIT	Gastrointestinal tract
GMC	General Medical Council
GnRH	Gonadotrophin-releasing hormone
GP	General Practitioner
GPI	General paralysis of the insane
G6PD	Glucosa 6 phosphate dehydrogenase
GTN	Glyceryl trinitrate
GIIb/IIIa	Glycoprotein IIb/IIIa (receptor)
GU	Genito-urinary
GUM	Genito-urinary medicine
Hb	Haemoglobin
HB Alc	Glycosylated haemoglobin
HBV	Hepatitis B virus
HCG	Human chorionic gonadotrophin
HCO3−	Bicarbonate
Hct−	Haematocrit
HCV	Hepatitis C virus
HDL	High density lipoprotein
HELLP	Elevated liver enzymes and low platelet count
HIB	*Haemophilus influenzae* type B (vaccine)
HIV	Human immunodeficiency virus
HLA	Human leucocyte antigen
HONK	Hyper-osmolar non-ketotic (coma)
HR	Heart rate
HRT	Hormaone replacement therapy

HSV	Herpes simplex virus
IBD	Inflammatory bowel disease
ICP	Intra-cranial pressure
IDDM	Insulin dependent diabetes mellitus
Ig	Immunoglobulin
IgM	Immunoglobulin M
IGT	Impaired glucose tolerance
IHD	Ischaemic heart disease
Im	Intramuscular
IMB	Intermenstrual bleeding
INR	International ratio
IOL	Induction of labour
IQ	Intelligence quotient
ISMN	Iso-sorbide mono-nitrate
ITU	Intensive therapy unit
IUCD	Intrauterine contraceptive device
IUGR	Intrauterine growth retardation
IV	Intravenous
IVP	Intravenous pyelogram
IVF	Invitro fertilisation
IVU	Intravenous urogram
K$^+$	Potassium
Kg	Kilogramme
KPa	Kilopascals
KUB	Kidneys/ureters/bladder
L	Litre
LDL	Low density lipoprotein
LFT	Liver function tests
LGV	Lymphogranuloma venereum
LH	Luteinising hormone
LHRH	Luteinising hormone releasing hormone
LKM-1	Liver, kidney, Muscle
LLETZ	Large Loop Excision of the Transformation Zone
LMN	Lower motor neurone
LMW	Low molecular weight
LNMP	Last normal menstrual period
LSCS	Lower segment caesarean section
MAOI	Mono-amine oxidase inhibitor
MCH	Mean corpuscular haemoglobin
MCP	Meta-carpophalangeal
MCV	Mean corpuscular volume
Mg++	Magnesium

MI	Myocardial infarction
mmol	Millimoles
MMR	Measles-mumps-rubella (vaccine)
MMSE	Mini mental state examination
Mph	Miles per hour
MRI	Magnetic resonance imaging
MS	Multiple sclerosis or Mitral stenosis
MSU	Mid stream urine
Na^+	Sodium
NAD	No abnormality detected
NEC	Necrotising enterocolitis
Neut	Neutrophilis
NG	Neoplasia (new growth)
NHL	Non-Hodgkin's lymphoma
NIDDM	Non insulin dependent diabetes mellitus
NSAID	Non steroidal anti-inflammatory drug
NSU	Non-specific urethritis
O2	Oxygen
OA	Osteoarthritis
OCP	Oral contraceptive pill
Od	Omni die (once daily)
OGD	Oesophagogastroduodenoscopy
OSCE	Objective structured clinical examination
PA	Postero-anterior
$PaCO_2$	Arterial pressure of carbon dioxide
PaO_2	Arterial pressure of oxygen
PAN	Perinuclear anti-neutrophilic
Panca	Perinuclear anti-neutrophilic cytoplasmic antibody
PCO	Polycystic ovaries
PCOS	Polycystic ovary syndrome
PCP	Pneumocystis carinii pneumonia
PCR	Polymerase chain reaction
PCV	Packed cell volume
PDA	Patent ductus arteriosus
PE	Pulmonary embolism
PEA	Persistent electrical activity
PEFR	Peak expiratory flow rate
PET	positron emission tomography
pH	Puissance d'Hydrogen = $-$ log (H+)
PICU	Paediatric intensive care unit
PID	Pelvic inflammatory disease
Plats	Platelets

PMH	Previous medical history
PND	Paroxysmal nocturnal dyspnoea
PNS	Peripheral nervous system
PO4$^-$	Phosphate
PPH	Post partum haemorrhage
PPI	Proton pump inhibitor
PR	Per rectum
PRHO	Pre-registration house officer
PRN	Pro re nata (as required)
PSA	Prostatic specific antigen
PT	Prothrombin time
PV	Per vagina
RBC	Red blood count
RCT	Randomised, controlled trial
Retics	Reticulocytes
ROM	Range of movement
RTA	Road traffic accident
RTA (I–IV)	Renal tubular acidosis
SACD	Subacute combined degeneration of the spinal cord
SAH	Subarachnoid haemorrhage
SARS	Severe acute respiratory syndrome
SCC	Squamous cell carcinoma
SDH	Subdural haemorrhage
SHBG	Sex hormone binding globulin
SIADH	Syndrome of inappropriate antidiuretic hormone secretion
SLE	Systemic lupus erythema
SOL	Space occupying lesion
SROM	spontaneous rupture of membranes
SSRI	Selective serotonin reuptake inhibitors
STEMI	ST elevation MI
STI	Sexually transmitted disease
Substance P	Vasoactive peptide and sensory neurotransmitter found in nerve cells and specialist gut endocrine cells SVT Supraventricular tachycardia
SVD	Spontaneous vaginal delivery
SVT	Supraventricular tachycardia
SXR	Skull X-ray
T3	Tri-iodo – thyronine
T4	Tetra – iodo -thyronine (thyroxine)
TB	Tuberculosis
TBM	Tuberculous meningitis
Tds	Ter die sumendus – (to be taken three times daily)

TED	Thrombo-embolic
TFTs	Thyroid function tests
T Helper	Thymus (lymphocytes)
TKco	Transfer coefficient
TIA	Transient ischaemic attack
TOP	Termination of pregnancy
TPA	Tissue plasminogen activator
TPHA	Treponema pallidum haemagglutination assay
TSH	Thyroid stimulating hormone
TT	Thrombin time
TVM	Transvaginal monitoring
U&Es	Urea and electrolytes
UMN	Upper motor neurone
Ur	Urea
USS	Ultrasound scan
UTI	Urinary tract infection
UV	Ultra violet
UV prolapse	Utero-vaginal prolapse
VDRL	Venereal disease research laboratory
VMA	Vanillylmandelic acid
V/Q scan	Ventilation/perfusion scan
VSD	Ventricular septal defect
V-V Fistula	Vesico-vaginal fistula
VZV	Varicella zoster virus
WCC	White cell count

Normal Values

In the majority of OSCE data interpretation stations it is customary in undergraduate examination to provide a set of normal values. Please refer to the list below when attempting any of the data interpretation stations in all three volumes of OSCEs.

Haematology

Haemoglobin

	Males	13.5 – 17.5 g/dl
	Females	11.5 – 15.5 g/dl

MCV	76 – 98 fl
PCV	35 – 55%
WCC	4 – 11 x 10^9/l
Neut.	2.5 – 7.58 x 10^9/l
Lymph.	1.5 – 3.5 x 10^9/l
Plt	150 – 400 x 10^9/l
ESR	0 – 10 mm in the 1st hour
PT	10.6 – 14.9 s
PTT	23.0 – 35.0 s
TT	10.5 – 15.5 s
Fib	125 – 300 mg/dl
Vitamin B_{12}	160 – 900 pmol/l
Folate	1.5 µg/l

Ferritin

	Males	20 – 250 µmol/l
	Females	10 – 120 µmol/l

Immunoglobulins

IgM	0.5 – 2.0 g/l
IgG	5 – 16 g/l
IgA	1.0 – 4.0 g/l

Biochemistry

Na^+	135 – 145 mmol/l
K^+	3.5 – 5.0 mmol/l
Urea (ur)	2.5 – 6.5 mmol/l
Cr	50 – 120 µmol/l
ALT	5 – 30 iu/l
AST	10 – 40 iu/l
Bili.	2 – 17 µmol/l
Alk Phos	30 – 130 iu/l
Albumin	35 – 55 g/l
αGT	5 – 30 iu/l

αFP	< 10 ku/l
CCA^2	2.20 – 2.60 mmol/l
PO$_4{}^{2-}$	0.70 – 1.40 mmol/l
CK	23 – 175 iu/l
LDH	100 – 190 iu/l
Amylase	< 200 u/l
Lactate	0.5 – 2.2 mmol/l
Mg^{2+}	0.75 – 1.00 mmol/l
Urate	0.1 – 0.4 mol/l
CRP	0 – 10 mg/l

Diabetes

Glucose		
	Random	3.5 – 5.5 mmol/l*
	Fasting	< 7 mmol/l
HbA1c		< 7.0%

Endocrinology

TSH		0.17 – 3.2 mu/l
fT$_4$		11 – 22 pmol/l
fT$_3$		3.5 – 5 pmol/l
Cortisol		
	0900	140 – 500 nmol/l
	2400	50 – 300 nmol/l
Growth hormone		< 10 ng/ml
Cholesterol		< 5.2 mmol/l
Triglycerides		0 – 1.5 mmol/l
LDL		< 3.5 mmol/l
HDL		> 1.0 mmol/l
Total/ HDL		< 5.0
FSH		1 – 25 u/l
LH		1 – 70 u/l
Prolactin		< 400 mu/l

Blood gases

pH	7.35 – 7.45
pA (CO$_2$)	4.6 – 6.0 kPa
pA (CO$_2$)	10.5 – 13.5 kPa
HCO$_3{}^-$ (bicarbonate)	24 – 30 mmol/l
BE	–2 – 2.0 mmol/l

CSF

Protein	< 0.45 g/l
Glucose	2.5 – 3.9 mmol/l (two-thirds plasma)
Cells	< 5 (WCC)
Opening pressure	6 – 20 cmH$_2$O

* If >5.5 then OGTT 2 h: 7 – 11.1 = IGT

                                               > 11.1 = DM

Generic approach to examinations

As with all OSCE stations, clinical examination stations should have clear, precise candidate instructions. **Read them carefully before starting** (and before asking any questions!) and if you are still unclear as to what you are being asked to do, clarify the task with the examiner.

For all clinical examinations you should try and follow the five steps given below. Some examinations may require you to modify or vary these stages:

1 **Introduction and consent**
2 **Observation and comment**
3 **Palpation**
4 **Auscultation**
5 **Presentation of findings and differential diagnoses or causes**

1 Introduction and consent

- Introduce yourself to the patient: with your name and role
- Explain what you would like to do and obtain verbal consent for the examination, eg 'I am just going to listen to your heart sounds, 'is that alright?' or 'Would it be alright if I examine your chest, legs'
- Keep these requests simple and in lay terms. Avoid medical jargon such as 'I would like to examine your peripheral nervous system' or 'would it be alright if I examine your cranial nerves?' Better to ask 'Would it be alright if I examine the function of your arms or legs' or ' Would it be alright if I examine the function of the nerves that control your face?'

2 Observation and comment

- Stand at the **END** of the patient's bed and comment on relative positives and negative manifestations. Look for relevant signs and they will be there – If you fail to look for them, they may not appear!
- Do not just say 'I'm looking for...'. **Comment** on the presence or absence of relevant signs
- Move back to the patient's right-hand side, re-clarify before starting your examination if you should start at the hands (if not stated in the instructions)
- **Look** for relevant signs – **comment** on their presence/absence.
- BUT expect to be challenged on findings/causes of anything you mention.

3 Palpation

- Be sure you have washed your hands in warm water before commencing any the examination. There is usually an alcohol wash at the bedside of each patient, which you should use between stations. If not, you should wash your hands between each patient, but be careful you do not leave the examiner behind, as he or she might be a little irritated.

- Whenever palpating:
  - (i) Reassure the patient before starting
  - (ii) Watch the patient's face for distress at all times
  - (iii) Apologise if any distress is caused
  - (iv) If distressed before the start of the examination – suggest appropriate analgesia.

4 Auscultation

- Understand what the stethoscope and its components are for, ie how to use the bell and the diaphragm (Bell = Low frequency) and even which way round to put the earpieces in your ears!
- Always tap the piece (bell or diaphragm) you are about to place on the patient with a finger, thus ensuring it is orientated the correct way. This saves 'no sounds heard': embarrassing silence!
- Always make sure the stethoscope pieces are warm (like you hands) before placing them on the patient.
- Your stethoscope should hang so the bell/diaphragm lies just below your waistline. This means you may need to cut longer tubes down but be wary of cutting off too much!
- With the more expensive/sophisticated stethoscopes you will hear sounds more easily and clearly. However, you may wish to buy a mid range one first to learn the basics.
- Know how to use the stethoscope, if you choose to buy an expensive/sophisticated one.

As with all the examination techniques, palpation, ballotting, auscultation and percussion, practice makes perfect! Initially you may feel more comfortable practising in the clinical skills laboratory on manikins and normal people, however **you must** practice in the various clinical settings on patients with and without clinical signs. Essential parts of the examination cannot be practised on friends and mannequins. Overcoming embarrassment or anxieties, talking and interacting with patients and relatives and, most importantly, recognising when patients are ill and eliciting clinical signs. At the end of every examination make sure you cover the patient up and thank them. Take every opportunity to examine patients, checking appropriate subjects with housemen and your peers, but make sure you have permission from the patient and the sister-in-charge.

5 Presentation of clinical findings, differential diagnoses and causes.

- Your presentation should be simple and concise. Present relevant positives and negatives, a differential diagnosis or causes.
- If you know the diagnosis, present the positive findings to support your diagnosis.
- 'This well looking, middle-aged man has signs consistent with aortic stenosis as evidenced by his low volume pulse which was slow rising in character. He has a narrow pulse pressure and his apex beat is hyperdynamic but undisplaced. On auscultation he has a grade 4/6 ejection systolic murmur heard loudest in the aortic area and radiating to the carotids. He has no signs of heart failure and no stigmata of endocarditis'.
- If you do not know the diagnosis, present the relevant positive and negative findings in a concise, logical manner. The simplest way to achieve this is to present the evaluations in the order of your examination, ie start at the hands, work up the forearm, the arm (including blood pressure), the face and neck, chest, abdomen and other regions of interest.
- 'This well looking middle-aged man had no peripheral stigmata of cardiovascular disease. His pulse was 72 bpm and regular, it was symmetrical and I was unsure but I think the character was abnormal. His blood pressure was 110/100 but I couldn't see his jugular venous pulse. His carotids were easily felt and had an abnormal character, although I couldn't define it. The apex beat was undisplaced and forceful. He had no heaves or thrills. On auscultation he had a systolic murmur heard loudest in the aortic area and I think it radiated to the carotids and the mitral area. He had no pulmonary or peripheral oedema. In summary, I think he may have aortic stenosis'.
- At the end of your presentation you should present a list of the common differentials or causes of the patient's problem.
- The examiner may challenge you on anything that you state, eg if you say the patient has clubbing, you might be asked some causes of clubbing.
- As with all clinical skills, presentation of findings and differentials requires practice.

Chapter 1:
Paediatrics

Contents

Chapter 1

Paediatrics

Paediatric History

When you take a paediatric history, discuss first what is of concern. Use the lists below to find out more about the area of concern, for instance the antenatal, birth and development in a child with fits. Go beyond these questions in an area of interest. There are too many questions here to ask in every situation, but touch on each area. For instance, 'are there any problems with his heart?' can be used rather than asking about scans and murmurs. **The most important aspect of history taking is to listen**.

Pregnancy

Planned/unplanned/IVF/donor/adopted
Scans – when and any problems
Previous births – gestation and weight
Mode of delivery – induction/SVD/LSCS (emergency or elective), and why
Resuscitation needed
SCBU afterwards
Apgars (but parents unlikely to know)

Development

Any concerns
Problems at school – academically or in games
Developmental screen (only use in < 5 years unless developmental problem):

Smiling	by	6 weeks (time of concern)
Sitting	by	9 months
Turns to sound	by	6 months
First words	by	18 months
Walking	by	18 months
Talking two-word sentences	by	3 years

Growth

Weight at birth

Any problems

Smaller than friends?

Immunisations

Up to date

Immunisation schedule	2, 3, 4 months – DTP, HIB, MenC, Polio
	12–14 months – MMR
	4 years – DT, Polio, MMR
	12 years – BCG

Who is at home?

Full family tree, with ages

Consanguinity

Any childhood deaths – more questions

Ask specifically about atopy/epilepsy/congenital heart disease/diabetes

Previous medical history

Sees GP – for what

Seen at hospital outpatients and why

Any hospital admissions, emergency or elective and why

Social

Housing – ask if any problems

Who looks after children – nanny/au pair/grandparents?

Ask if any involvement with social services; be tactful?

Income support

Parental employment

Pets if allergic or infectious problem.

Respiratory

Any breathing difficulties

How is he now

Noisy breathing – inspiratory or expiratory

Episodes of cyanosis, apnoea or working hard

What makes it better/worse

Day or night variation

Cough – dry/wet/barking, worse at night

Previous treatments and their effect

Cardiovascular

Antenatal scans

Murmur heard – how investigated?

Episodes of cyanosis or shortness of breath, especially feeding

Operations?

Gut and nutrition

Breastfeeding – any problems. Is baby satisfied by feed, how often?

Milk – which formula, how much, how often?

Concerns about growth – (look at 'centiles in red book)

Eating solids (after about 4 months)? Any dietary requirements

Diarrhoea/constipation – consistency, how often – any treatment

Vomiting – what/when/how much

Take a 24 h intake/output history

Renal

Previous UTIs – any investigations

Unexplained fevers

Irritability/blood in urine

Swelling around eyes or abdomen.

Bones and joints

Any problems running?

Swollen joints

Neurological

How are they doing at school? – development

Any fits – if so, age, type, investigations, medication used

Interventions

Medications and inhalers, special diets

STATION 1.1

Examination

You are the paediatric PRHO in an outpatient clinic. You have been asked to see a 6-week-old baby with a murmur. Having taken a full history, you now come to the examination. Please demonstrate to the examiner how you would examine a child with this problem.

(5 minute station)

STATION 1.2

Examination

You are the paediatric PRHO in the Emergency Department. A 10-year-old girl with asthma presents with breathing difficulties. She has already had a salbutamol nebuliser. Please assess her respiratory system.

(5 minute station)

STATION 1.3

Abdominal examination

Please examine this 5-year-old's abdomen. His mother has said that his abdomen is becoming more distended.

(5 minute station)

STATION 1.4

Growth

Michael has been attending the growth clinic. Please can you measure his growth and plot them on a centile chart fig 1.4a. The examiner may then ask you some questions based on this. Please use any of the equipment provided in fig 1.4b.

(10 minute station)

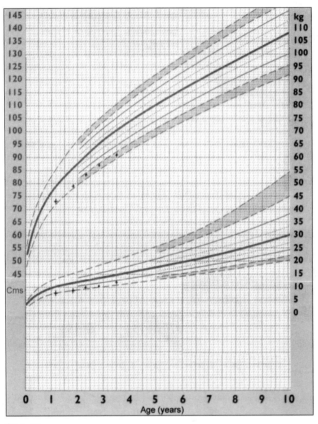

fig 1.4a

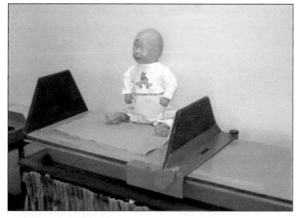

fig 1.4bi

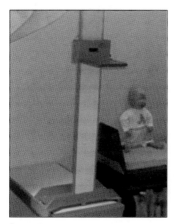

fig 1.4bii

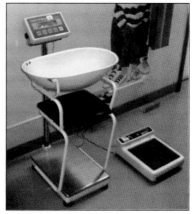

fig 1.4biii

STATION 1.5

Examination of the Head

Please demonstrate to the examiner how you might examine this baby's cranium.

(5 minute station)

STATION 1.6

Dysmorphology examination
Please examine this 4-year-old child with a possible genetic condition.

(5 minute station)

STATION 1.7

Neurology examination
Please examine the limbs of this 5-year-old boy.

(5 minute station)

STATION 1.8

Developmental examination
You are the doctor in a child development clinic. Rory has come for his 9-month check. Please assess his development.

(10 minute station)

STATION 1.9

Skin examination

Look at the five images (figs 1.9a, 1.9b, 1.9c, 1.9d, 1.9e) of various skin appearances. Please complete the following table by selecting one of the available diagnoses and management plans. Each diagnosis and plan can be used once, more than once, or not at all.

(5 minute station)

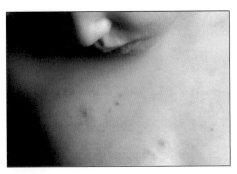

fig 1.9a

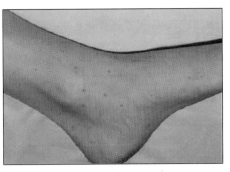

fig 1.9b

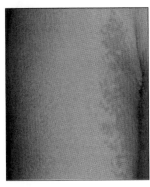

fig 1.9c

fig 1.9d

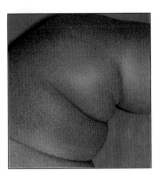

fig 1.9e

Meningococcal sepsis

Herpes simplex

Chickenpox

Rubella

Molluscum contagiosum

Milaria

Capillary haemangioma

Cavernous haemangioma

Eczema

Café au lait patch

Pityriasis versicolor

(Mongolian) blue spot

Reassure – it will resolve spontaneously

Reassure – it is a birthmark

Systemic aciclovir

Topical aciclovir

Surgery

Dietary advice

Topical antifungal

Systemic steroids

Topical steroids

Observe

Intravenous antibiotics

Picture	Diagnosis	Management plan
fig 1.9a		
fig 1.9b		
fig 1.9c		
fig 1.9d		
fig 1.9e		

STATION 1.10

Examination of gait
Please watch this 7-year-old boy walk and comment on what you see. Then please demonstrate additional clinical signs that you think are relevant.

(5 minute station)

STATION 1.11

Newborn examination
You are the neonatal SHO. Please demonstrate and talk the examiner through how you would examine this 4-day-old baby. He was born after an uneventful pregnancy and normal delivery. He is now breastfeeding well.

(10 minute station)

STATION 1.12

Growth faltering/social history
You are a general practitioner. Mrs Robinson has come to see you because she is concerned about her child's poor growth. Please take a history with a view to making a diagnosis. You will be asked to summarise this at the end and suggest a management plan.

(15 minute station)

STATION 1.13

Convulsion history

You are the paediatric SHO. You have been asked to see a child who has had a fit and been brought into the Emergency Department by his mother. Please take a history, and then be prepared to discuss the diagnosis and management plan.

(15 minute station)

STATION 1.14

Respiratory History

Alfie has been brought into the Emergency Department by his parents because they are concerned about his coughing. Please take a history and be prepared to discuss your management plan.

(15 minute station)

STATION 1.15

Abdominal history

You are the surgical House Officer. The casualty officer has referred you a 9-month-old boy who has been vomiting with what appears to be a painful abdomen. Please take a history and make an assessment based on this.

(15 minute station)

STATION 1.16

Presentation of fever

Table 1.16 contains five histories typical of children with various infectious illnesses. Arranged in a haphazard manner with these are organisms and a diagnosis. Please rearrange the organisms and diagnoses so they match the presentation.

(5 minute station)

Patient History	Organism	Diagnosis
1 A 6-year-old child with a fever, a convulsion and altered consciousness	(A) *Escherichia coli*	(a) Septicaemia
2 A 6-year-old with a low grade fever, a cough and an erythematous rash	(B) *Neisseria meningococcus*	(b) UTI
3 A 6-month-old girl with a temperature of 40°C, irritability, cardiovascularly stable.	(C) Haemophilus influenzae	(c) Otitis media
4 A child with reduced consciousness, a purpuric rash and a low blood pressure.	(D) Herpes simplex	(d) Chest infection
5 An infant of 9 months with irritablity, fever, pulling at his ear.	(E) *Mycoplasma*	(e) Encephalitis

Table 1.16

Answers

1 (   ) (   )

2 (   ) (   )

3 (   ) (   )

4 (   ) (   )

5 (   ) (   )

STATION 1.17

Presentation of Vomiting

In Table 1.17 are five histories of children with vomiting. Along with these, but arranged in a haphazard manner, are five causes and management strategies. Please rearrange the diagnoses and management plans to match the presentation.

(5 minute station)

Patient History	Causes	Management plan
1 A girl of 8 weeks has been vomiting large amounts of altered milk after every feed for the last 6 weeks but is otherwise well.	(A) Pyloric stenosis	(a) Oral rehydration
2 A girl of 9 months has a temperature of 38.5°C and intermittent vomiting. She also has watery diarrhoea.	(B) Gastrooesophageal reflux	(b) Urgent operation
3 A boy of 7 weeks presents with an increasingly frequent non-bilious vomiting and dehydration.	(C) Possetting	(c) Observe and reassure
4 A boy of 3 days becomes acutely unwell with abdominal distension, bilious vomiting and hypotension	(D) Gastroenteritis	(d) Feed thickeners
5 After every feed a 4-week-old-baby brings up small amounts of milk on to and around his chin.	(E) Volvulus	(e) Fluid resuscitation then operation

Table 1.17

Answers

1 (   ) (   )

2 (   ) (   )

3 (   ) (   )

4 (   ) (   )

5 (   ) (   )

STATION 1.18

Neonatal Cardiopulmonary Resuscitation

You are the neonatal PRHO attending the delivery suite. After a long labour a baby boy is delivered by forceps for fetal distress. The baby is placed on the resuscitaire for you to manage. The baby is apnoeic, asystolic, white and unresponsive. Please demonstrate what you would do with the model. Some equipment is provided in fig 1.18.

(5 minute station)

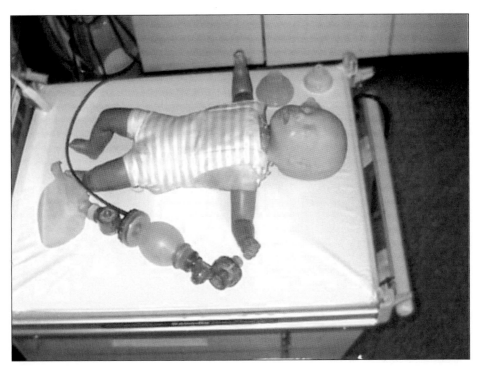

fig 1.18

STATION 1.19

Paediatric airway

You are the casualty SHO. Brought in by blue light ambulance is a 5-year-old known epileptic. He had a generalised tonic clonic seizure at home. He was given 2 mg rectal diazepam by his parents and then another 2 mg rectal diazepam by the ambulance staff to stop his seizure. This was successful but he has now stopped breathing. His pulse is 120, saturations 80% in face mask oxygen. Please demonstrate with the model how you would manage him using the equipment provided (fig 1.19).

(5 minute station)

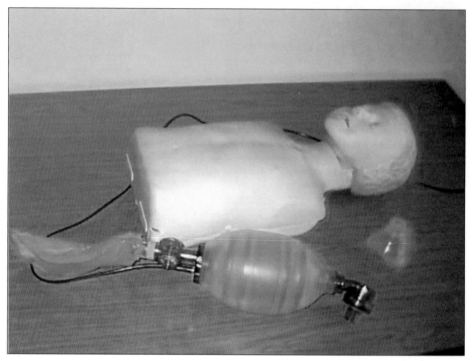

fig 1.19

STATION 1.20

Respiratory explanation

Maddy is a 2-year-old girl who is now ready for discharge from the paediatric ward following an acute asthma attack. She has a long history of nocturnal cough and one previous admission. You are the paediatric SHO. Using the equipment provided (fig 1.20) and the prescription, part of which is shown below, please explain to Maddy's mother how to use the medicine.

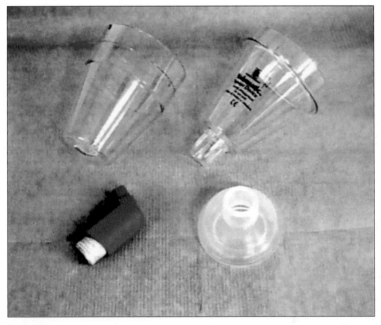

fig 1.20

Drug name	Dose	Frequency	Days supply	Duration	Pharmacy
Beclomethasone via spacer	100 mcg	bd	2 weeks	to continue	
Salbutamol via spacer	100 mcg	qds/prn	2 weeks	to continue	
Volumatic spacer device					

(5 minute station)

STATION 1.21

Respiratory explanation

Markus is 7 years old and he was diagnosed with asthma at age 2. He gets attacks when the weather is damp and has exercise-related wheeze. He takes 2 x 100 mcg puffs of Becotide beclomethesone via a spacer twice a day and salbutamol 100 mcg as required. Please can you demonstrate to him how to use the peak flow device supplied (fig 1.21), and explain to him and his mother what to do with the readings.

(10 minute station)

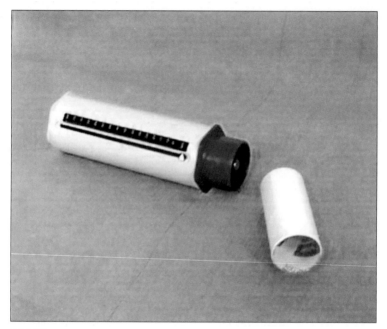

fig 1.21

STATION 1.22

Therapeutics

Isobel is a 5-month-old girl of 7.2 kg. She had been in hospital for the last 3 days because of high fever, irritability and diarrhoea. After a full septic screen, she was found to have a urinary-tract infection. This is the final report on the clean catch urine specimen.

(10 minute station)

PATHOLOGY			MICROBIOLOGY
Name 1	**Name 2**	**Unit Number**	**Date of Birth**
Isobel	Walters	VR148295	03/08/03
Ward	**Consultant**	**Date sent**	**Time sent**
Rocket	JECR	02/02/04	09.06

Specimen type clean catch urine

Microscopy	Culture	Sensitivity/Resistance	
RBC 15	$E.COLI > 10^8$	AMPICILLIN	R
WBC >200		CEPH	S
NO ORGANISMS SEEN		TRIMETHOPRIM	S
		CIPROFLOXACIN	S
		GENT	S

Isobel was initially treated with IV cefotaxime and made a good recovery. She is now ready for discharge and has her follow-up arranged. The consultant has asked you to arrange her medicines to take home. Please can you prescribe these using the prescription form provided and the *British National Formulary* at the station.

First name _____   **Second name** _____

Date of Birth ____-____-____   **Unit number** _____

Drug Name	Dose	Frequency	Days supply	Duration	Pharmacy

Prescriber's name _____ **Signature** _____ **Date** ____-____-____

fig 1.22

STATION 1.23

Explanation of results

Mark's mother has come to see you for the results of his investigations. Two weeks ago he was seen for his poor weight gain and several investigations were sent off – a full blood count, urea, electrolytes and liver function, clean-catch urine, all of which were within normal limits. The report on the other investigation is below. Please look at the investigation and explain to the mother what it means.

PATHOLOGY			*BIOCHEMISTRY*
Name 1	**Name 2**	**Unit Number**	**Date of Birth**
Mark	Gates	VS025632	13/9/03
Ward	**Consultant**	**Date sent**	**Time sent**
POPD	JECR	31/01/04	12.34

Investigation	Sweat test
Sweat weight	46 g
Sweat chloride	95 mmol/l
Comment	Insufficient sweat volume

(10 minute station)

STATION 1.24

Explanation

You are the doctor in a child health clinic. The health visitor asks you to see a 3-month-old baby with her mother. The mother is worried about the next set of immunisations that are due today.

(10 minute station)

STATION 1.25

Paediatric explanation – asthma

Connor is a 3-year-old who has come to you, his GP, for a follow-up visit. He was admitted to the local hospital with an acute asthma attack. He was discharged and an appointment made to see you 6 weeks later. His mother has brought the following letter:

Dear GP,

Connor O'Connell was admitted to hospital on 12/9/03 and discharged on 14/9/03 with an acute exacerbation of asthma. He was initially treated with nebulised salbutamol and oral prednisolone and made a good recovery. He was discharged on inhaled salbutamol, 100 mcg qds. Follow-up will be with the GP at 6 weeks to review the medication.

Yours,

(10 minute station)

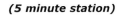

STATION 1.26

Investigation – Chest Radiograph

Please look at the chest radiograph in fig 1.26 taken from a preterm newborn with difficulty in breathing. Please name the structures marked.

(5 minute station)

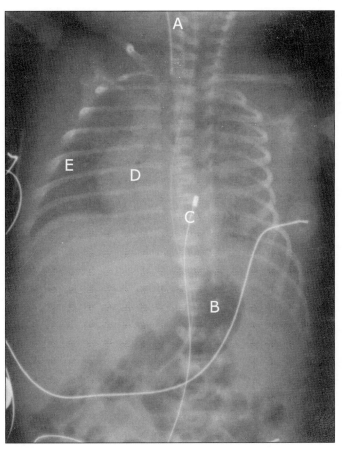

fig 1.26

A

B

C

D

E

STATION 1.27

Paediatric investigations

Summer is a 3-month-old girl who has had several chest infections and is not gaining weight appropriately. She is tachypnoeic with subcostal recession. This radiograph has been taken as part of her assessment. Please look at the radiograph in fig 1.27 and report it to the examiner and then suggest a management plan.

(5 minute station)

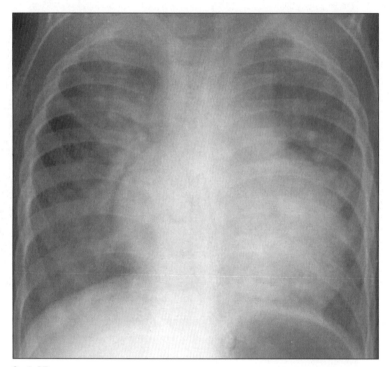

fig 1.27

STATION 1.28

Paediatric investigations

Michael is a 3-month-old boy being investigated for a urinary-tract infection. The investigation shown in fig 1.28 is part of this. Please look at the investigation and explain what it shows to the examiner.

(5 minute station)

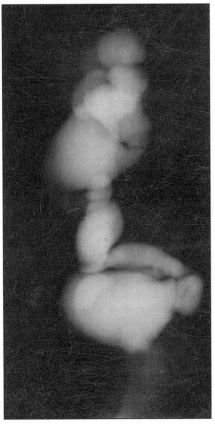
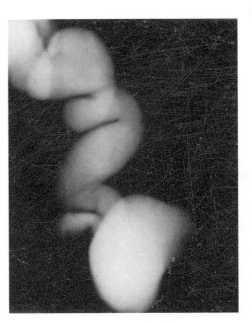

fig 1.28

STATION 1.29

Paediatric ECG

Look at the ECG in fig 1.29 taken from a newborn infant. Describe the ECG to the examiner; then explain how you would assess the baby.

(5 minute station)

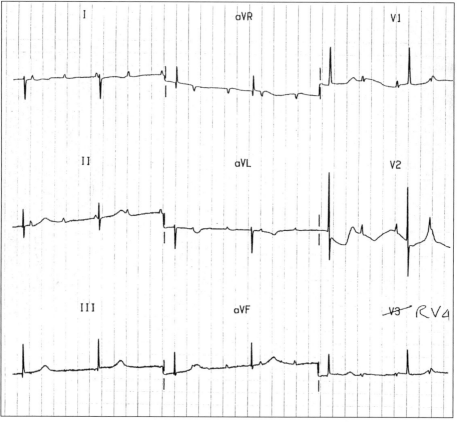

fig 1.29

STATION 1.30

Paediatric radiology and management

Please look at the chest radiograph in fig 1.30 from a 4-week-old baby boy. His parents have brought him to the Emergency Department because of concern about his cough and fast breathing. He has been feeding poorly for the last 2 days.

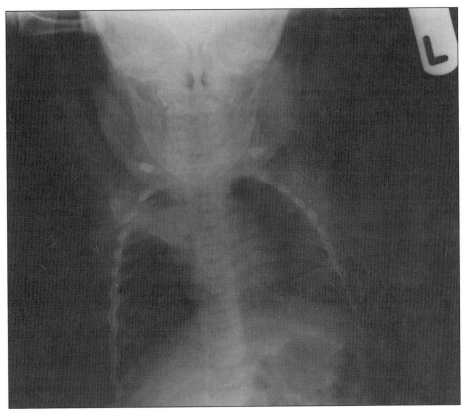

fig 1.28

HR 170

RR 70

SaO$_2$ 82% in air.

The examiner will now ask you some questions based on this information.

(10 minute station)

Chapter 2:
Obstetrics and Gynaecology

Contents

Obstetric and gynaecological histories

Obstetrics and gynaecology examinations

Chapter 2

Obstetrics and Gynaecology

Obstetric and Gynaecological Histories

Obstetric history

- **Previous pregnancies**
  Number
  Successful deliveries
  Miscarriages
  Abortions – spontaneous and planned terminations
  A full-term pregnancy is regarded as 40 weeks, with the duration of the pregnancy written as a division of this, eg pregnancy of 22 weeks and 3 days is written $\dfrac{22+3}{40}$

- **Number of children and ages**
  Gravidity, G, describes the number of times a woman has been pregnant. Parity, P, describes the number of pregnancies that have proceeded after 28 weeks (x) and those that terminated before (y), ie P = x+y. A woman who has had two terminations, two miscarriages before 28 weeks and one full term delivery, and who is now expecting her second child is described as G6, P1+4.

- **Antenatal problems**
  Hypertension
  Diabetes
  Heart disease
  Polyhydramnios
  Intrauterine death
  Family history/previous history of multiple pregnancies

- **Method of delivery**
  Normal vaginal delivery
  Forceps/vacuum extraction
  Caesarean section

- **Birth weight**

- **Perinatal problems**
  Mother and baby
  Congenital abnormalities
  Antenatal/postportum haemorrhage
  Last normal menstrual cycle/period (LNMP)
  Last sexual intercourse
  Fertility treatment
  Methods of contraception/pregnancy planning

- **Symptoms of early pregnancy**
  Amenorrhoea
  Breast engorgement
  Nausea and vomiting (hyperemesis gravidarum)
  Associated urinary symptoms

- **Feelings of patient and partner about pregnancy**

Gynaecological history

Menarche: age of onset of menstruation, usually between 10 and 16 years old.

Normal menstrual cycle:

Duration of menstrual bleeding	eg	_5_ days
Duration from start of one normal menstruation to the start of the next		25

Dysmenorrhoea: painful periods.

Menorrhagia: heavy menstrual bleeding defined by the number of days of bleeding, number of towels and tampons used, volume of blood and clots passed.

Polymenorrhagia: frequent heavy bleeding.

Oligomenorrhoea: infrequent menstruation.

Amenorrhoea: absence of menstruation > 6 months; this may be primary or secondary. Primary applies to girls who have not menstruated by 16. Secondary applies to female patients who have experienced menstruation which has subsequently stopped.

Causes of amenorrhoea

Hypothalamic: Kallman's syndrome (isolated LHRH deficiency).

Pituitary: prolactinoma – large pituitary tumours causing loss of pituitary function, or those interfering with the pituitary stalk causing hyperprolactinaemia.

Ovarian: polycystic ovary syndrome, premature ovarian failure.

Vaginal: imperforate hymen, vaginal stenosis.

General: anorexia nervosa, severe illness, testicular feminisation, thyroid dysfunction, endurance athletes, eg marathon and triathletes.

Intermenstrual bleeding: may be secondary to infection, cervical polyp or carcinoma.

Post-coital bleeding: causes include cervical erosion/infection, trauma and malignancy.

Vaginal discharge: physiological, infective, erosive or neoplastic. Nature and duration and association with menstrual cycle or intercourse.

Vaginal bleeding: physiological, erosive, neoplastic, menstrual abnormalities, post-coital.

Cervical smear: last smear date, result, family history of cervical carcinoma.

Premenstrual syndrome (PMS): this is a cyclical pattern of symptoms experienced by a woman prior to menstruation. Common symptoms include bloating, breast tenderness, irritability, labile mood, fluid retention and headache.

Sexual history: includes number of partners and sexual contacts, contraceptive methods, terminations of pregnancies (abortions), sexually transmissible diseases/pelvic inflammatory disease.

Dyspareunia: pain on sexual intercourse; may be superficial, because of local infection or atrophic vaginitis, or deep, because of pelvic inflammatory disease or endometriosis.

Menopause: this is when a woman stops menstruating for at least 6 months. There is often a period around this time when a woman will have infrequent periods and suffer with symptoms of increased oestrogen deficiency. This is known as the climacteric. Symptoms include hot flushes, palpitations and atrophic vaginitis. Symptoms of oestrogen deficiency are improved by hormone replacement therapy, which also reduces the risk of developing atherosclerotic disease and osteoporosis.

Post-menopausal bleeding: this must be regarded as carcinoma of the endometrium until proven otherwise.

Obstetrics and Gynaecology Examination

Gynaecological examination

Abdominal palpation for pelvic masses or tenderness.

Bimanual pelvic examination.

Speculum examination should precede digital examination if there is a history of vaginal discharge or bleeding.

Obstetric examination

Symphysis-fundal height in centimetres, after 20 weeks should correspond to the period of amenorrhoea.

Determine fetal position (lie and presentation) at near term and auscultate the fetal heart rate.

Vaginal examination only when indicated; it should never be performed 'routinely'.

STATION 2.1

History

A 27-year-old woman sees you, her GP, on the first antenatal visit. Please take her history.

(5 minute station)

STATION 2.2

History

A 29-year-old woman seeks an urgent consultation with you, her GP. She is worried that she may be pregnant. Please take a relevant gynaecological history.

(5 minute station)

STATION 2.3

History

The same patient as in Station 2.2 is found to have a positive pregnancy test. Please counsel her on her pregnancy, and elicit her underlying concerns.

(5 minute station)

STATION 2.4

Please read through the following information before attempting the next station.

(5 minute station)

You are the House Officer attached to an obstetric and gynaecology firm. The next patient is a 24-year-old primigravida at 28 weeks gestation who is returning to the antenatal clinic 1 week after a routine oral glucose tolerance test screening, the results of which are shown below.

Glucose tolerance test

Ms. Phoebe Oxley DOB 13.01.79

Unit no. 098456

Fasting 6.8 mmol/l (ref <7.0)

120 min–12.5 mmol/l (ref 7–11 impaired glucose tolerance

> 11.1 = gestational diabetes)

STATION 2.4a

Explanation

The 25-year-old primigravida is attending the antenatal clinic today for the results of her glucose tolerance test. Please explain the results, implications and management to the patient.

(5 minute station)

STATION 2.5

Preparatory

Please read through the following information before attempting the next station.

(5 minute station)

STATION 2.5a

You are a medical student attached to a general practitioner. The next patient is 34 weeks pregnant and is under shared care between the hospital and the GP. She has been under review because of her blood pressure as shown below.

CWD = consistent with dates; NAD = no abnormality detected

Date	Week	Fundal height	BP	Urinalysis
12 April	32^{+4}	CWD	120/70	NAD
17 April	33^{+2}	CWD	140/90	NAD
22 April (today)	34^{+2}	CWD	157/98	Protein ++

Please explain the implications of today's blood pressure and urinalysis for her and her baby and the immediate management you think should be followed.

(5 minute station)

STATION 2.6

History

You are a PRHO working in the antenatal clinic. The next patient is a 24-year-old primigravida who had a routine ultrasound at 20 weeks gestation which showed a low lying placenta. Yesterday she had a repeat scan at 34 weeks gestation, which showed the placenta lying anteriorly in the lower segment and completely covering the cervical os. Please explain the ultrasound findings to her and the future management.

(5 minute station)

STATION 2.7

History

A 20-year-old primigravida wishes to discuss pain relief during her prospective labour. You are a medical student at the antenatal clinic – please discuss the analgesic options available to her.

(5 minute station)

STATION 2.8

Examination

Please perform an abdominal examination on this antenatal patient and explain your findings to the examiner as you proceed.

After this, the examiner will ask you the following question:

- What other checks would you perform at an antenatal examination?

Equipment provided:

A 'pregnant' manikin, sphygmomanometer, fetal stethoscope.

(5 minute station)

STATION 2.9

Investigation

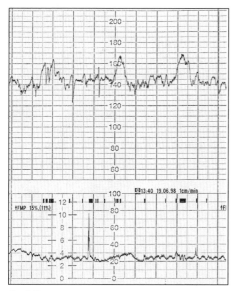

fig 2.9a

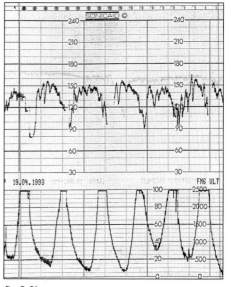

fig 2.9b

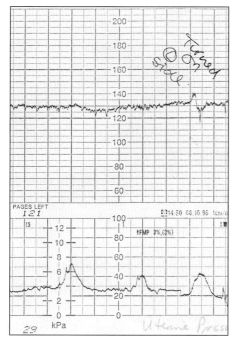

fig 2.9c

Figs 2.9a, 2.9b and 2.9c are fetal cardiotacographs (CTGs) taken during labour in a 27-year-old primigravida. Comment on the normal and abnormal (if present) components of each of the tracings and give one underlying factor that may produce the changes.

(5 minute station)

STATION 2.10

Examination

Please complete the following table of Apgar scores of the newborn infant.

(5 minute station)

Apgar Scores

	0	1	2
Colour			
Heart rate			
Respiratory effort			
Muscle tone			
Reflex response			

STATION 2.11

Examination

Please perform a clinical examination of the newborn baby (represented by a manikin) to detect any abnormalities that may have been missed soon after birth.

(5 minute station)

STATION 2.12

Treatment

Please demonstrate on the model, using the equipment provided, the resuscitation procedure in a neonate born in an asphyxiated condition.

(10 minute station)

Materials provided:

Manikin for neonatal cardio-respiratory resuscitation
Resuscitation (tilt) trolley
Piped 100% oxygen and suction source, face mask, ambu-bag and tubing
Oro-pharyngeal intubation set
Heart rate monitor
Sodium bicarbonate ampule, with 2 ml syringe, venous IV catheter set
Mechanical ventilator
Blankets, heating pad.

STATION 2.13

History

You are a medical student attached to a gynaecology outpatient clinic. The next patient is a 19-year-old student, who has been referred by her GP for amenorrhoea. Please take a history of the presenting complaint and any further relevant history and give an appropriate diagnosis to the examiner.

(5 minute station)

STATION 2.14

History

A married couple have come to see you, their GP, with difficulty in starting a family. Please take a history from the wife with a view to assessing their fertility problems. You may assume she is alone on this visit.

(10 minute station)

STATION 2.15

History

A 33-year-old woman is referred to the gynaecological clinic by her GP for sterilisation. Please take a history to assess her request.

(5 minute station)

STATION 2.16

Explanation

A 35-year-old, single woman consults you, her GP, with period pain. Please take a relevant history with a view to making an appropriate diagnosis.

(5 minute station)

STATION 2.17

History

A 45-year-old woman consults you, her GP, with a history of heavy menstrual bleeding. Please take a relevant history and tell the examiner an appropriate diagnosis.

(5 minute station)

STATION 2.18

History

You are a medical student. A 27-year-old woman is referred to the gynaecology clinic (where you are working) complaining of a vaginal discharge which, despite the GP's reassurance, continues to trouble her. Please take an appropriate history, with a view to making a diagnosis.

(5 minute station)

STATION 2.19

History

Please read the following information before attempting the next station.

You are a medical student attached to a general practitioner's surgery. The next patient is a 34-year-old woman who has returned to see the GP for the results of a cervical smear which she has recently had and was reported:

'Severely dysykaryotic squamous cells with enlarged nuclei consistent with a diagnosis of CIN III. A colposcopy is advised.'

Please explain the cervical smear report to the patient and the future management involved.

You do NOT need to take a history from her.

(5 minute station)

STATION 2.20

History

A 58-year-old woman consults you, her GP, complaining of a dragging sensation in her vagina. Please take an appropriate history.

The examiner will ask you for a diagnosis at the end.

(5 minute station)

STATION 2.21

Examination

Please carry out a bimanual examination on the pelvic manikin, explaining your actions to the observer as you proceed. You are not required to perform a smear test or pass a speculum. You do not need introduction, explanation or consent.

(5 minute station)

STATION 2.22

Examination

Please perform a cervical smear on a pelvic manikin using the appliances provided in fig 22.2. You should explain your actions to the observer as you proceed.

(5 minute station)

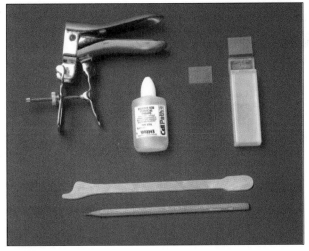

fig 2.22

STATION 2.23

Investigation

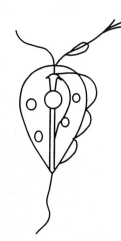

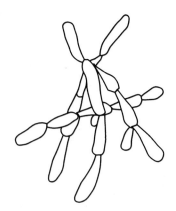

fig 2.23a   fig 2.23b

A 31-year-old woman complains of vaginal irritation and discharge. She was found to be infected by organisms as shown in figs 2.23a and 2.23b.

1 Name the organisms shown in figs 2.23a and 2.23b.

2 How would you arrive at an immediate diagnosis?

3 State your treatment measures for figs 2.23a and 2.23b.

4 What factors predispose to infection with these pathogens.

(5 minute station)

STATION 2.24

Investigation

Fig 2.24 was obtained as part of the investigation of a 33-year-old woman at the fertility clinic.

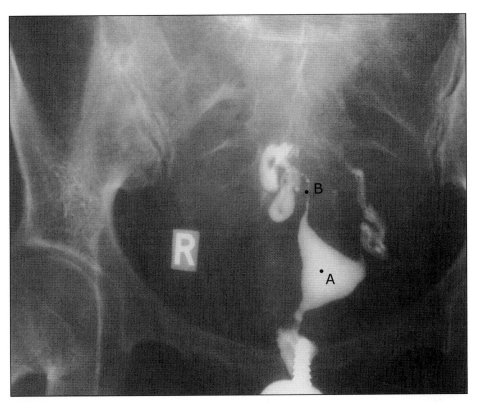

fig 2.24

1 Name the investigation performed.
2 State two clinical conditions that may show abnormalities with this investigation.
3 Identify the structures labelled A and B.
4 How is this investigation performed?
5 State one other option available to make a similar assessment.

(5 minute station)

STATION 2.25

Investigation

A 33-year-old woman was found to have human chorionic gonadotrophin (HCG) levels in excess of 100 000 IU/l in her urine following a miscarriage at 20 weeks.

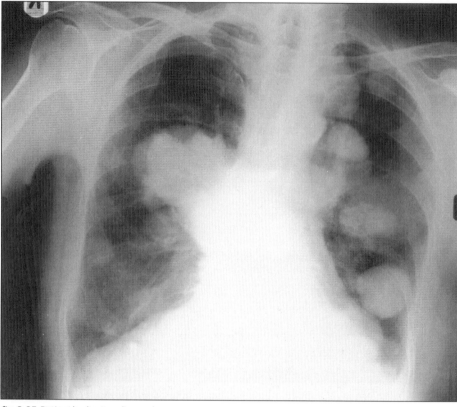

fig 2.25 Patient's chest radiograph

1 State three causes of excessively elevated urinary HCG levels during or following pregnancy.
2 State the positive finding on the radiograph and your diagnosis.
3 How would you treat this patient?

(5 minute station)

STATION 2.26

Examination

Please perform a breast examination on the manikin provided and tell the examiner what you are doing as you go along.

Equipment – Breast exam manikin

(5 minute station)

STATION 2.27

History

You are a medical student attached to an obstetrics firm. The next patient is a 25-year-old who is attending the antenatal clinic for her first visit of this pregnancy. The consultant has asked you to see her before he does. Please take a history of her current pregnancy, her previous obstetric history and any relevant gynaecological history.

(5 minute station)

STATION 2.28

Explanation

You are a medical student on a clinical placement in the Family Planning Clinic. A 21-year-old student has come in today and discussed contraception with the doctor. The doctor has asked you to explain to her how to put on a condom and what to do if it breaks. Equipment required: condom in packet and condom trainer.

(5 minute station)

STATION 2.29

Information-giving

You are a medical student attached to a general practice. The GP has asked you to see this 24-year-old lady who has come to the surgery today to discuss starting the combined oral contraceptive pill for the first time. Please advise her on how to take a combined oral contraceptive pill and any appropriate information to ensure good compliance (and hence contraception). You do not need to take any further history from her.

(10 minute station)

STATION 2.30

Explanation

You are a medical student attached to an obstetrics firm. The next patient is a 25-year-old bank clerk who is currently 16 weeks in her first pregnancy. She is attending the antenatal clinic after her serum screening for Down's syndrome gave a high-risk result of 1:80 (age-related risk 1:1500). The consultant has asked you to see her as she has decided to have an amniocentesis and would like to discuss this test further. Please counsel her with regard to the procedure. You do NOT need to take her history.

(10 minute station)

STATION 2.31

Investigation and explanation

You are a medical student attached to an obstetrics firm. The next patient is a 25-year-old bank clerk who is currently 34 weeks gestation in her first pregnancy. She is attending the antenatal clinic after an ultrasound. Her midwife had felt that she was clinically small for dates with a symphysis-fundal height of 29 cm. Inform her of the significance of the ultrasound findings and what may happen in terms of her management over the next few days and weeks. Her BP and urinalysis have always been normal.

(5 minute station)

Ultrasound report:

Gestation = $34^{+2}/40$

Singleton pregnancy

Fetal heart = present 145 bpm

Placenta = Anterior not low

Liquor volume = reduced (amniotic fluid index AFI = 66 mm)

Umbilical Doppler = +ve but reduced end diastolic flow

Growth

HC = Head circumference

AC = Abdominal circumference

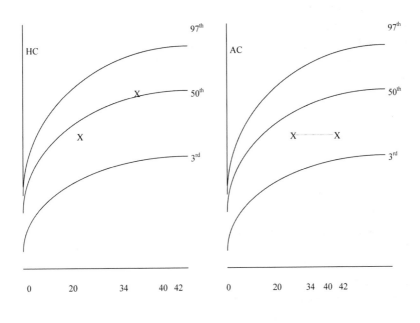

fig 2.31 Ultrasound report

STATION 2.32

Investigation

Look at figs 2.32a, 2.32b, and 2.32c and answer the corresponding questions below.

(10 minute station)

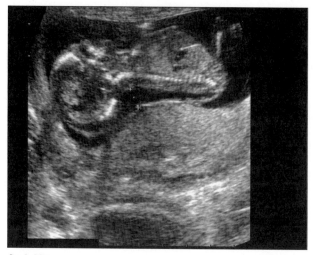

fig 2.32a

1 This ultrasound image was taken at 11-14 weeks. What measurement is used at this stage to assess gestational age?
2 What measure do the callipers show?
3 Name one clinical abnormality that this test may screen for.
4 Give two diagnostic options that are available to parents in this circumstance.

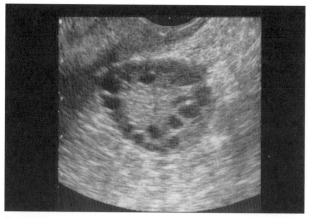

fig 2.32b

5 Which organ is demonstrated here and what abnormality does it show?

6 Name three clinical features that may be associated with this finding

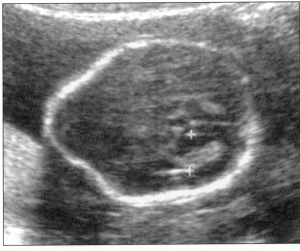

fig 2.32c

7 What abnormality is seen here?

8 What causes this abnormality?

9 What can be done to prevent this from occurring?

STATION 2.33

Instruments

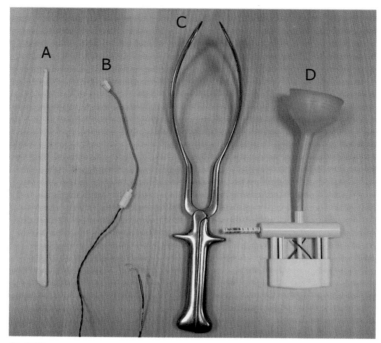

fig 2.33

1 Name A and give two indications for its use.
2 Name B and give one indication for its use.
3 Give five prerequisites before the instruments C and D may be used.
4 Name three complications that may occur with use of D.
5 Which of C or D is the recommended instrument of choice for operative delivery?

(10 minute station)

Chapter 3:
Endocrine and Breast

Contents

Chapter 3

Endocrine and Breast

Endocrine and Diabetes Mellitus History

Endocrine disorders often present with multiple, non-specific symptoms and it is, therefore, important to take a precise history. Many are autoimmune in nature and it is important to establish whether patients have a family history of endocrine and autoimmune disease.

General symptoms linked to endocrine disease

- **Malaise**:
  Lethargy and lassitude

- **Weight loss**:
  Thyrotoxicosis
  Type 1 DM
  Adrenal malignancy

- **Weight gain:**
  Hypothyroidism
  Cushing's (centripetal obesity)

- **Menstrual irregularity:**
  Prolactinoma
  Thyroid disease
  Polycystic ovary syndrome
  Hypopituitarism

- **Male impotence:**
  Prolactinoma
  Hypopituitarism
  IDDM

- **Proximal muscle weakness/wasting:**
  Cushing's disease
  Thyrotoxicosis
  Acromegaly

- **Sleeping problems**:
  Somnolence (hypothyroidism)

- **Loss of libido:**
  Hypopituitarism
  Gonadal failure

- **Mood:**
  Depression
  Poor concentration (hypothyroidism)

- **Pigmentation**
  Particularly buccal, skin creases and scars (Addison's disease)

- **Acne and hirsutism:**
  Cushing's syndrome
  Polycystic ovary syndrome
  Adrenal malignancy
  Congenital adrenal hyperplasia

Specific symptoms of endocrine disease

- **Pituitary disease:**
  Local symptoms: headache, visual disturbances (classical bitemporal hemianopia).
  Systemic symptoms: classified according to the disorder; functioning and non-functioning pituitary tumours.

- **Acromegaly:**
  Coarsening and enlargement of facial features.
  Overbiting mandible, with increased interdental separation.
  Enlargement of hands, feet and head circumference; shoes, gloves and hats do not fit.
  Proximal limb girdle weakness.
  Symptoms of hypertension and diabetes mellitus
  Visceromegaly: may lead to cardiac failure and hepatosplenomegaly.

- **Prolactinoma:**
  Galactorrhoea
  Spontaneous expression of milk from the nipples.
  Oligo/amenorrhoea.
  Female infertility; male impotence; loss of libido in both sexes.

- **Cushing's disease:**
  Proximal myopathy with centripetal obesity.
  Abdominal striae.
  Symptoms of hypertension and diabetes mellitus.

- **Hypopituitarism:**
  Patients may present in a very non-specific manner with symptoms of thyroid, gonadal and adrenal insufficiency.

Diabetes

Diagnostic symptoms

Polyuria: passing large volumes of urine.

Polydypsia: increased thirst.

Increased infections: UTIs, candidiasis.

Weight: older type 2 DM patients are often overweight.

Younger type 1 DM patients often lose weight before diagnosis.

Patients often complain of non-specific symptoms, such as malaise and lethargy.

Complications

These should be well defined in the history, particularly in established disease.

Macrovascular: IHD, stroke, PVD.

Microvascular: retinopathy and nephropathy.

Neuropathic: peripheral sensory neuropathy ('stocking and glove' distribution).

Mononeuritis multiplex: this is multiple nerve palsy with no apparent anatomical association, eg oculomotor, median and lateral peroneal palsies.

Autonomic: may present with postural hypotension or male impotence.

TIAs and CVAs.

Others: it is important to specifically ask about foot and eye problems, particularly visual acuity and foot ulceration.

Diabetic control

Method of testing: BM stix or urinalysis, frequency; results.

Compliance with diet.

Weight.

Method of control: diet only; tablets; insulin regimen.

Follow-up: diabetic liaison nurses, GP, hospital frequency.

OSCE Stations

Risk factors

It is essential to address the associated risk factors for diabetic complications.

Smoking.

Dietary: excess fat and refined sugar must be excluded; dietician review.

Alcohol excess: among many other problems, alcohol contains a lot of calories.

Hypertension.

Hyperlipidaemia: diabetes causes hypertriglyceridaemia.

Obesity: excess fat causes increased insulin resistance.

Thyroid examination and assessment

For OSCE and other clinical assessment purposes examination of the thyroid is often divided into:

(a) Examination of the thyroid mass/goitre

(b) Assessment of the patient's thyroid status.

In clinical practice they may often be combined.

Examination of the thyroid mass/goitre

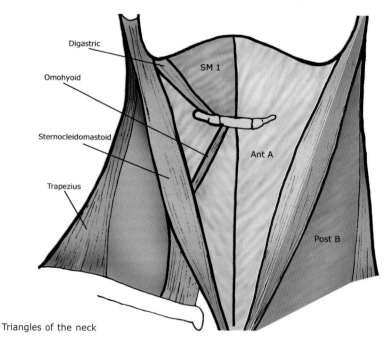

Triangles of the neck

1 Site.

2 Size.

3 Shape.

4 Surface.

5 Consistency.

6 Attachments (superficial and deep).

7 Bruits.

8 Transillumination.

9 Check for associated lymphadenopathy.

Note

a With a midline neck mass, check for movement with protrusion of the tongue. A thyroglossal cyst will move superiorally or 'upwards' with protrusion of the tongue.

b With a large goitre – check for retrosternal extension by percussing over manubrium of the sternum.

Specific examination for thyroid swelling

Patient should be seated:

1 Observe patient's neck from anterior position. Note site, size, shape of neck mass; look for other signs of thyroid disease (see thyroid status).

2 Ask patient to take a sip of water – 'hold it in your mouth':

- observe mass as patient is asked to swallow

- thyroid mass should 'rise and fall' with swallowing.

3 Now palpate mass from behind patient. Defining the nine characteristics above; repeat the swallow assessment while palpating thyroid mass from behind.

4 Complete examination by defining/excluding:

- thyroid bruit

- retrosternal extension (only if you cannot define its lower border).

Assessment of thyroid status

As with all examinations it is easiest to remember these features by the order in which you examine them, ie from the hands upwards.

	Hyperthyroidism (thyrotoxicosis)	Hypothyroidism
Hands	Onycholysis Sweaty palms Palmar erythema Fine tremor	Cold, dry peripheries
Pulse	Tachycardia (resting)	Bradycardia
Upper limbs	Proximal myopathy	
Eyes	Lid lag	
Face/hair		Loss of outer third of the eyebrows; dry hair, 'peaches and cream' complexion; 'toad-like facies'
Thyroid	Bruit	
Reflexes	Brisk	'slow-relaxing'
General	Thin, agitated	Overweight, depressed, mentally slow, poor concentration (can present in coma!)

Both may be associated with a goitre and have features of Graves' triad, which is made up of:

- Thyroid acropachy (pseudo clubbing)
- Graves' eye signs (orbitopathy) – exophthalmos/ptotosis/cranial nerve palsies (III, IV, VI); lid retraction, nystagmus
- Pre-tibial myxoedema.

Breast examination

Examination of the breasts is a potentially embarrassing examination for both medical student and patient. It is important that you have examined real patients and not made do with the simulation and protective environment of the clinical skills department. Part of the examination is how you deal with the intimate nature of this situation; how you attempt to place the patient at ease; and how you confront your own anxieties. It is also essential when performing an intimate examination on a member of the opposite sex that you have a chaperone with you at all times.

Start your examination by introducing yourself with name and role. Explain the examination and ask permission to continue. You will need to adequately expose both breasts and ask the patient to remove her bra. However, you should leave the patient covered with a blanket or dressing gown until you need to examine the breasts. This is very important to maintain the patient's dignity and keep them at ease. If the patient presents with a mass ask them to point out its position.

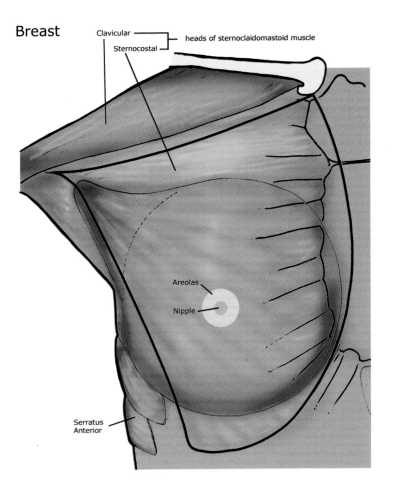

Breast
Clavicular
Sternocostal — heads of sternoclaidomastoid muscle
Areolas
Nipple
Serratus Anterior

Observation: look for symmetry of size and shape of the breasts, areolas and nipples. Note any dimpling of the skin or obvious masses.

Palpation: it is important to reassure the patient your hands are clean and warm before starting to palpate the breast. With the breast supported by your non-dominant hand firmly but gently palpate the four quadrants of each breast, examine the areaolae and nipples. If a mass is palpable you will need to define its characteristics and examine for axillary, supraclavicular and cervical lymphadenopathy. Specifically examine for fixity to the deep muscle layer by asking the patient to place their hands on their hips and squeeze (testing for fixity to the pectoralis muscles) and place their hands behind their head (testing for fixity to the pectoralis major muscle)

Sinister features of a breast mass include:

- Tethering to deep and superficial structures
- Recent inversion of the nipple
- Bloody discharge from the nipple
- Ulceration of the overlying skin
- Dimpling of the skin (known as peau d'orange = skin of an orange)
- Hard, immobile, irregular shape
- Bilateral masses
- Associated lymphadenopathy
- Associated hepatomegaly
- Associated bone pain (percuss lumbar spine)

STATION 3.1

History

You are a medical student attached to an endocrinology firm. The next patient is a 25-year-old man, who has been referred by his GP with a worsening frontal headache and complaining that his shoes and gloves have become too small for him. Please take a history of the presenting complaint with a view to making a diagnosis.

(10 minute station)

STATION 3.2

History

You are the House Officer on a general medical and endocrine firm. The next patient is a 21-year-old woman who has been referred by the gynaecologists with a history of irregular periods. Please take a history of the presenting complaint, including a gynaecological history, with a view to making a diagnosis.

(10 minute station)

STATION 3.3

History

You are the medical student attending endocrine outpatients. The next patient is a 34-year-old woman, who has been referred by her GP for weight gain, striae and bruising. Please take a history of the presenting complaint with a view to making a diagnosis.

(5 minute station)

STATION 3.4

History

You are the medical student attending endocrine outpatients. The next patient has been referred by the gynaecologists, with irregular periods, hirsutism and obesity. Please take a history of the presenting complaint with a view to making a diagnosis. You should include a full gynaecological history.

(5 minute station)

STATION 3.5

History

You are the medical student attached to a general medical firm. The next patient is a 54-year-old woman, who has been referred to outpatients with a croaky voice and weight gain. Please take a history of the presenting complaint and any other relevant history with a view to making a diagnosis.

(5 minute station)

STATION 3.6

History

You are a medical student attending the diabetes clinic. The next patient is a 54-year-old man who has had type 2 DM for the last 10 years. He has come in today for a review appointment. Please take a history to establish this gentleman's diabetic control. Screen for possible complications.

(10 minute station)

STATION 3.7

History

You are the House Officer attached to a general medical firm. You have been asked to take a history from a 21-year-old woman with malaise, lethargy, a random blood glucose, taken by her GP, is 35.6 mmol/l. You should concentrate on the presenting complaint and associated relevant history, and be prepared to discuss the future management of this patient.

(10 minute station)

STATION 3.8

History

You are the House Officer on a general medical firm. You have been asked by the registrar to explain the implications, treatment and possible complications of diabetes mellitus to a newly diagnosed 21-year-old patient.

(5 minute station)

STATION 3.9

History

You are a medical student attending the endocrinology clinic, when you are asked to obtain a history from a 30-year-old female, as depicted in fig 3.9. An actor may play the role of patient.

(5 minute station)

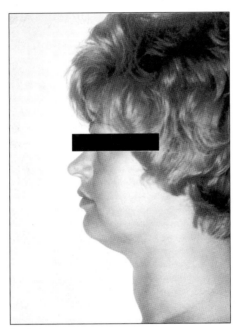

fig 3.9

STATION 3.10

Examination

Examine the neck of the patient whose history you have taken in the preceding station. Please make a full clinical assessment of this neck mass (do not assess the thyroid status).

(10 minute station)

STATION 3.11

Examination:

The patient you have just examined with a long-standing goitre complains of feeling anxious and unwell for the past few weeks. Please make an assessment of her thyroid status with a view to making a diagnosis.

(5 minute station)

STATION 3.12

Examination

Figs 3.12a and 3.12b are women with goitres.

(5 minute station)

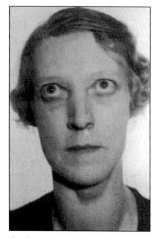

fig 3.12a

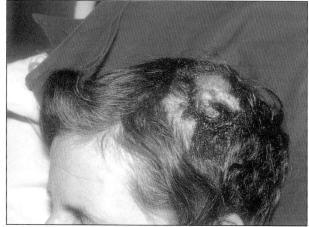

fig 3.12b

Questions

1 What are the probable diagnoses in each?

2 State one investigation that would confirm the diagnosis in both patients.

3 State the cause of the abnormality of the eyes in 3.12a and the swelling on the scalp in 3.12b.

4 State the principles of treatment for each patient.

STATION 3.13

Examination

(10 minute station)

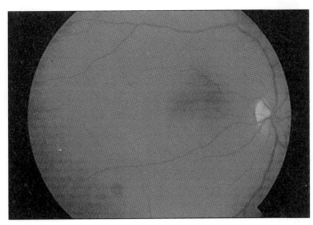

fig 3.13a

1 (fig 3.13a)	True	False
(a) There is evidence of hypertensive retinopathy.	☐	☐
(b) The macula shows evidence of senile degeneration.	☐	☐
(c) There is a blot haemorrhage in the upper temporal quadrant.	☐	☐
(d) There is evidence of papilloedema.	☐	☐
(e) There are some dot haemorrhages in the lower nasal areas.	☐	☐

OSCE Stations

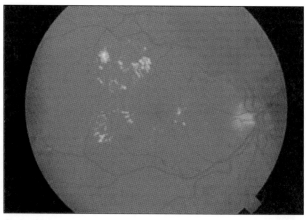

fig 3.13b

2 (fig 3.13b)	True	False
(a) There is evidence of macular damage.	☐	☐
(b) There is evidence of optic atrophy.	☐	☐
(c) There are soft exudes in the inferior nasal quadrant.	☐	☐
(d) There are hard exudates in the inferior nasal quadrant.	☐	☐
(e) This slide shows evidence of pre-proliferative diabetic retinopathy.	☐	☐

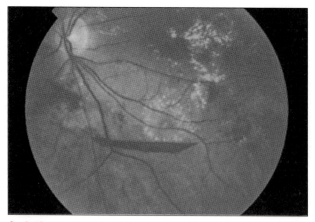

fig 3.13c

3 (fig 3.13c)	True	False
(a) There is a macular 'star' present.	☐	☐
(b) There is a subhyaloid haemorrhage.	☐	☐
(c) There are soft exudates in the inferior nasal quadrant.	☐	☐
(d) There are blot haemorrhages in the upper temporal quadrant.	☐	☐
(e) There is evidence of papilloedema.	☐	☐

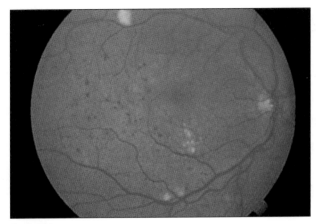

fig 3.13d

4 (fig 3.13d)	True	False
(a) The optic disc is normal.	☐	☐
(b) The macula is normal.	☐	☐
(c) There are soft exudates present.	☐	☐
(d) This patient has had previous laser therapy to the retina.	☐	☐
(e) The patient must be treated with insulin.	☐	☐

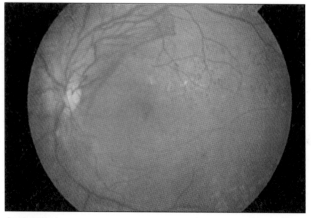

fig 3.13d

5 (fig 3.13e)	True	False
(a) There is evidence of neovascularisation.	☐	☐
(b) There is evidence of previous laser therapy in the superior and inferior temporal quadrants.	☐	☐
(c) This patient requires urgent ophthalmology review.	☐	☐
(d) There are multiple soft exudates present.	☐	☐
(e) There is evidence of optic atrophy.	☐	☐

STATION 3.14

Investigation
Please match the causes of hyponatraemia with the brief histories and diagnoses below.

(5 minute station)

Patient history	Diagnosis
1 A 29-year old man with a long history of steroid use now presents with postural hypotension and pigmented scars.	(a) Psychogenic polydypsia
2 A 64-year-old woman with a croaky voice, constipation and lethargy.	(b) Diuretic use
3 A 27-year-old man with a 6-day history of a dry cough, fever and malaise.	(c) Addison's disease
4 A 37-year-old woman drinking 6-7 litres of water per day. Blood glucose = 5.2mmol.	(d) Primary hypothyroidism
5 A 69-year-old man with biventricular cardiac failure.	(e) Atypical pneumonia with SIADH (syndrome of inappropriate secretion of antidiuretic hormone)

OSCE Stations

Answers

1 (   )

2 (   )

3 (   )

4 (   )

5 (   )

STATION 3.15

Investigation

The disorders listed below are associated with changes in serum potassium levels. Please list them under the correct headings.

(5 minute station)

Cushing's disease	Frusemide infusion	Acute renal failure
Addison's disease	Conn's syndrome	Lisinopril
Spironolactone	Type IV RTA	Ectopic ACTH secretion
Type I renal tubular ocidosis (RTA)	Fanconi's syndrome	Cardiac failure with secondary hyperaldosteronism

Hypokalaemia

(< 3.5 mmol/l)

Hyperkalaemia

(> 5.0 mol/l)

STATION 3.16

Investigation

Three diabetic patients arrive unconscious in the Emergency Department. Please calculate the osmolality and anion gap for each of the three patients and thus the type of diabetic coma each is suffering.

(refer to tables for normal values)

(5 minute station)

Plasma osmolality = 2 [Na^+ + K^+] +Ur +Glucose

      Normal range 280–295 mosmol/kg

Anion gap = [Na^+ + K^+] – [HCO_3^- + Cl-]

      Normal range 10–18 mmol/l

Patient A:

42-year-old woman

Medication: Metformin 850 mg bd

U+Es : Na+ 158 K+ 4.9 HCO_3^- 12 Cl- 102 Ur 34 Cr 162

      Glucose: 50 mmol/litre

      Lactate: 38.7 mmol/litre

      Urinalysis: Protein +++; Blood ++; Ketones ++

      MSU: Organisms +++

Patient B:

26-year-old man

Medication: Mixtard insulin 36 units mane, 20 units nocte

U+Es: Na+ 145 K+ 4.0 HCO_3^- 8 Cl- 106 Ur 14 Cr 44

      Glucose: 45.3 mmol/litre

      Lactate: 3.2 mmol/litre

      Urinalysis: Protein – trace; Blood – nil; Ketones +++

      CXR: Right lower lobe pneumonia

Patient C:

79-year-old man

Medication: Gliclazide 80 mg bd, Metformin 850 mg bd

U+Es: Na+ 155 K+ 4.5 HCO_3^- 25 Cl- 110 Ur 19.0 Cr 205

Glucose – 80 mmol/litre

Lactate – 6.0 mmol/litre

Urinalysis; – Protein + Blood: nil Ketones ++

STATION 3.17

Investigation

Using the data in the table below, choose the correct diagnosis for patients (A) to (E).

(5 minute station)

Normal range:	TSH	0.3–3.5 mU/l
	Total serum T3	1.2–3.1 nmol/l
	Free serum T4	13–30 pmol/l

Patient	TSH/mU/l	T3/nmol/l	T4/pmol/l	Diagnosis
A	67.2	0.9	0.5	
B	0.05	8.5	52.3	
C	2.0	1.0	7.0	
D	0.05	39.1	15.5	
E	2.6	2.8	24	

Diagnoses

1 Thyrotoxicosis

2 T3 Thyrotoxicosis

3 Primary hypothyroidism

4 Euthyroid

5 Sick euthyroid

STATION 3.18

Investigation

The patients listed below have abnormal bone and/or calcium metabolism. Please rearrange the table to match the histories with the correct data and diagnoses.

(5 minute station)

Patient history	Corrected Ca^{2+}	PO$_4^-$	Alkaline phosphatase	Diagnosis
1 29-year-old Asian woman with proximal limb weakness	(A) 2.32	1.02	3033	(a) Osteoporosis
2 31-year-old Black woman from Missouri, USA, with lupus pernio	(B) 1.82	1.3	107	(b) Multiple myeloma
3 73-year-old woman with premature menopause, now presenting with back pain	(C) 3.45	1.02	421	(c) Paget's disease of the bone
4 71-year-old man with an enlarged skull, deafness and hip and back pain	(D) 2.25	0.76	135	(d) Pseudo-hypopara-thyroidism
5 81-year-old man with multiple lytic lesions of the skull and bony pain	(E) 1.65	0.57	678	(e) Sarcoidosis
6 16-year-old woman with low IQ, short stature and short 4th and 5th metacarpals	(F) 2.98	0.92	104	(f) Osteomalcacia

OSCE Stations

Answers

1 (   )

2 (   )

3 (   )

4 (   )

5 (   )

6 (   )

STATION 3.19

Investigation

Three patients are taking part in a study of polyuria. One has cranial diabetes insipidus, one psychogenic polydypsia and the third is the control. From the water deprivation test results below, match the patients to the correct diagnosis.

(5 minute station)

	Time (hours)	Plasma osmolality (mosmol/kg)	Urine osmolality (mosmol/kg)	Body weight (kg)
Normal ranges		280–295	350–900	
Patient A	0	290	232	65.7
	4	294	272	63.4
	8	296	300	61.2
After DDAVP		292	596	
Patient B	0	291	550	82.2
	4	289	702	81.6
	8	292	840	81.4
After (DDAVP)		293	850	
1 – deamino				
8 – Dorguinine vasoplessin				
Patient C	0	268	320	72.0
	4	284	424	71.5
	8	290	510	71.1
After DDAVP		291	523	

Answers

Patient A

Patient B

Patient C

STATION 3.20

Investigation

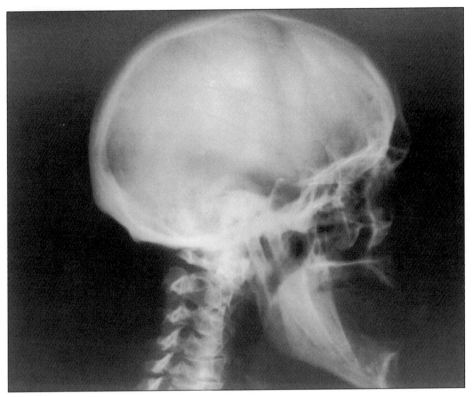

fig 3.20a

(5 minute station)

1 (fig 3.20a)	True	False
(a) This an AP view of the skull	☐	☐
(b) It shows lytic lesions	☐	☐
(c) The bony cortex is normal	☐	☐
(d) The sella is normal	☐	☐
(e) The appearances are consistent with acromegaly	☐	☐

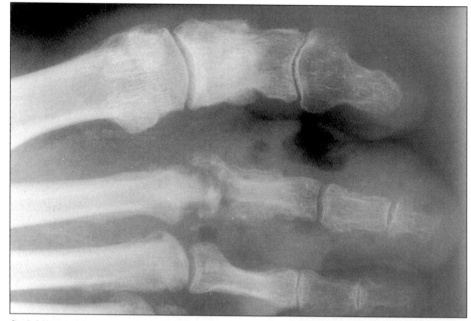

fig 3.20b

2 (fig 3.20b)	True	False
(a) This is a lateral radiograph of the foot	☐	☐
(b) There is calcification of the blood vessels	☐	☐
(c) The soft tissues are normal	☐	☐
(d) There is evidence of osteomyelitis	☐	☐
(e) The changes are suggestive of hyperparathyroidism	☐	☐

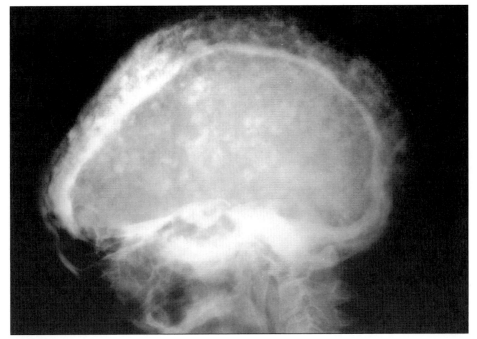

fig 3.20c

3 Fig 3.20c	True	False
(a) The bony cortex is thickened	☐	☐
(b) There are multiple lytic lesions	☐	☐
(c) There is platybasia	☐	☐
(d) The patient is at increased risk of developing optic atrophy	☐	☐
(e) The patient is at increased risk of developing an osteosarcoma	☐	☐

STATION 3.21

Investigation

Please indicate whether the statements regarding the radiographs shown below are **TRUE** or **FALSE**.

(5 minute station)

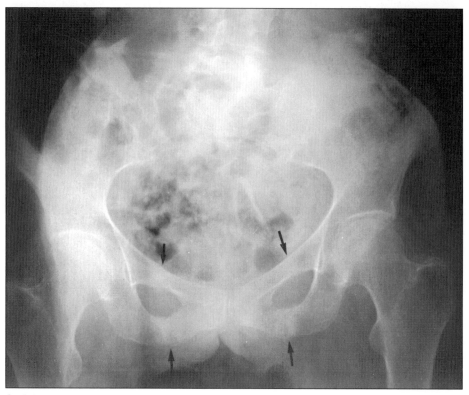

fig 3.21a

1 (fig 3.21a)	True	False
(a) This is a PA radiograph of the pelvis	☐	☐
(b) The bones are osteopaenic	☐	☐
(c) There is osteoarthritis of the right hip joint	☐	☐
(d) The patient's serum clacium will be greater than 3.0 mmol/l	☐	☐
(e) The alkaline phosphatase will be raised	☐	☐

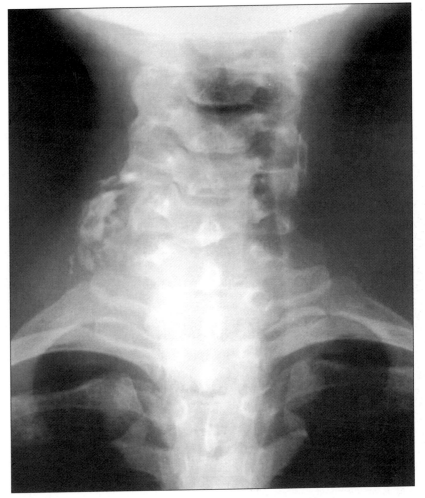

fig 3.21b

2 (fig 3.21b)	True	False
(a) This radiograph is a thoracic inlet view	☐	☐
(b) There is evidence of soft tissue swelling and calcification	☐	☐
(c) There is evidence of tracheal deviation	☐	☐
(d) There is a right-sided cervical rib	☐	☐
(e) These appearances are consistent with a calcified goitre	☐	☐

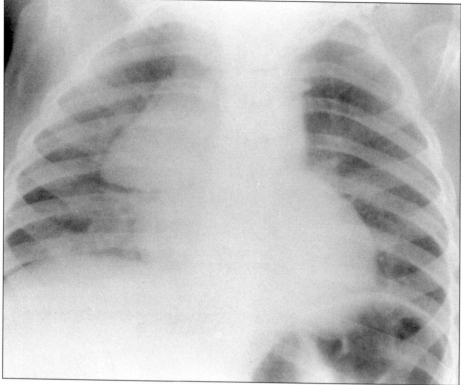

fig 3.21c

3 (fig 3.21c)	True	False
(a) This is an AP chest radiograph	☐	☐
(b) The patient is about 6 months of age	☐	☐
(c) The lungs fields are normal	☐	☐
(d) There is evidence of an aortic aneurysm	☐	☐
(e) This appearance is known as the 'sail' sign	☐	☐

STATION 3.22

Investigation

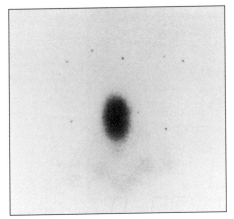

fig 3.22a

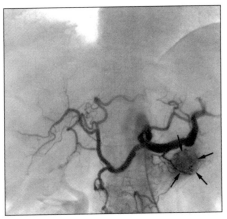

fig 3.22b

OSCE Stations

(5 minute station)

1 (fig 3.22a)

(a) What is this investigation?

(b) What does it show?

2 (fig 3.22b)

This patient presented with multiple blackouts and a recorded serum glucose of 2.0 mmol/l.

(a) What is this investigation?

(b) What do the arrows define?

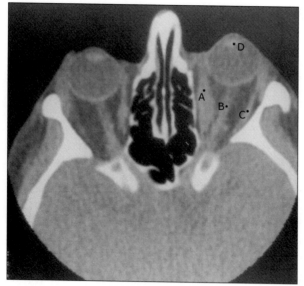

fig 3.22c

3 (fig 3.22c)

This is a CT scan taken through the orbits.

(a) Label the structures (A) to (D).

(A)

(B)

(C)

(D)

(b) What are the abnormalities?

(c) List two further clinical signs that are associated with these abnormalities.

(d) List two further investigations you would perform.

STATION 3.23

Investigation

A 37-year-old woman complaining of breathlessness on exertion and orthopnoea had a plain radiology of the thoracic inlet fig 3.23.

(5 minute station)

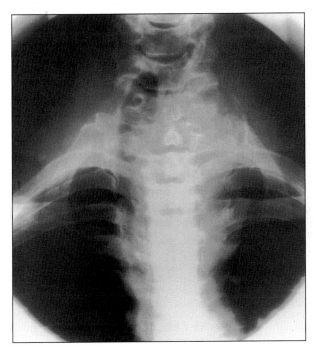

fig 3.23

1 What are the radiological findings?

2 What is the probable cause of her symptoms?

3 What radiographs would you request to further evaluate her symptoms?

4 State the definitive measure to relieve her symptoms.

STATION 3.24

Investigation
Please label structures A-G in the MRI scan of the pituitary fossa and surrounding
structures.

(5 minute station)

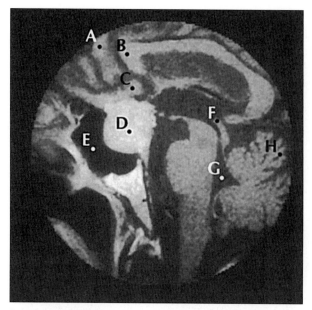

fig 3.24

(A)   (E)

(B)   (F)

(C)   (G)

(D)   (H)

Figs 3.24 and 3.25 are reproduced by kind permission of Prof J.P. Monson,
Consultant Endocrinologist, St Bartholomew's Hospital, London.

STATION 3.25

Investigation

Please label structures A–H in this the CT scan of the abdomen taken at the level of L2 – L3 shown in fig 3.25.

(5 minute station)

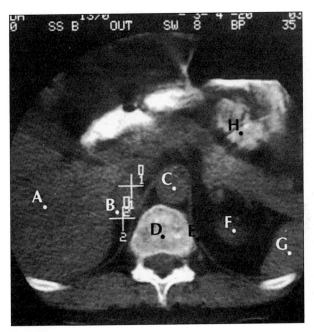

fig 3.25

(A)   (E)

(B)   (F)

(C)   (G)

(D)   (H)

STATION 3.26

Investigation

Fig 3.26 shows the thyroid gland in a 63-year-old euthyroid woman with a palpable nodule in the left lobe.

(5 minute station)

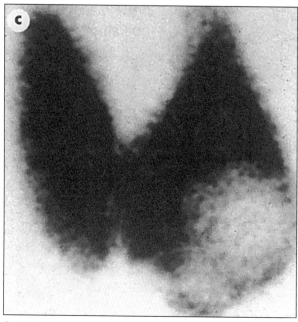

fig 3.26

1 State the imaging procedure shown and the agents used to obtain the scan.
2 Identify the site and nature of the abnormality on the scan. State three lesions that may be implicated.
3 What further investigations would be required to arrive at a definitive diagnosis?

Fig 3.26 from Besser GM, Thorner MO, ed *Atlas of Endocrine Imaging*, 1993, Mosby Europe Ltd Publishers. By Permission of Mosby International.

STATION 3.27

Therapeutics

You are a general practitioner new to this practice. Your next patient is a 48-year-old woman who believes she has recently started her menopause and has read in several magazines she should go on hormone replacement therapy. Please discuss the pros and cons of the treatment and establish whether she is a suitable candidate.

(5 minute station)

STATION 3.28

Therapeutics

Please match the diabetic treatments below to correspond with their correct side-effects and drug groups.

(5 minute station)

OSCE Stations

Drug	Drug group	Side-effect
1 Actrapid	(A) Sulphonylurea (t2 < 8 hours)	(a) Flatulence
2 Metformin	(B) Glucosidase inhibitor	(b) Lipoatrophy
3 Tolbutamide	(C) Short-acting insulin	(c) Alcohol-induced flushing
4 Acarbose	(D) Sulphonylurea (t2 > 24 hours)	(d) Lactic acidosis
5 Chlorpropamide	(E) Biguanide	(e) Hypoglycaemia

Answers

1 (   ) (   )

2 (   ) (   )

3 (   ) (   )

4 (   ) (   )

5 (   ) (   )

STATION 3.29

Therapeutics
You are a House Officer on a diabetes and general medical firm. You have been asked by your registrar to explain to a newly diagnosed 23-year-old diabetic patient how to draw up and inject insulin and to stress the important points of insulin therapy.

(10 minute station)

STATION 3.30

Therapeutics: Preparatory
Please read the following before attempting the next station.

Ms James is a 19-year-old nurse who recently underwent trans-sphenoidal surgery for a large pituitary tumour. This has left her panhypopituitary and she must remain on the treatments shown below until she is seen again in the outpatient department:

Thyroxine 100 mcg od

Hydrocortisone 20 mg mane; 10 mg nocte

Recombinant FSH/LH replacement

You should explain to the patient:

(a) The normal function of the pituitary gland hormones.
(b) The reason for using each of the above medications.
(c) The possible problems with the medications.

(5 minute station)

STATION 3.30a

Therapeutics
You are the House Officer of the endocrine firm looking after a 19-year-old nurse, who recently underwent hypophysectomy for a large pituitary tumour. You have been requested by the nursing staff on the ward to explain the nature and important points of her hormone replacement to the patient before she goes home.

(5 minute station)

STATION 3.31

History
You are a medical student in the breast clinic. Please take a history from this 34-year-old woman, who has been referred with incapacitating breast pain, with a view to making a diagnosis.

(5 minute station)

STATION 3.32

History
You are a medical student and the consultant has asked you to take a history from this 26-year-old woman seen at the breast clinic, who is anxious over the prospect of developing breast cancer because of a strong family history.

(5 minute station)

STATION 3.33

Examination

Fig 3.33. is that of a 43-year-old woman who attended the breast clinic for breast asymmetry since puberty. From your observations please state whether the following statements are correct.

(5 minute station)

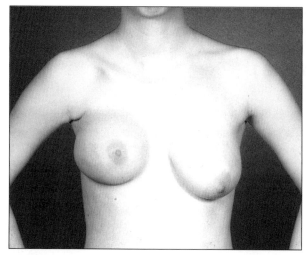

fig 3.33

	True	False
1 The patient has a problem with her self-image.	☐	☐
2 The right breast:		
(a) ptotic	☐	☐
(b) has developmental abnormality	☐	☐
(c) is cosmetically disfiguring	☐	☐
(d) cannot be corrected by breast enlargement.	☐	☐
3 The left breast:		
(a) has a normal contour	☐	☐
(b) has had a surgical procedure	☐	☐
(c) has nipple retraction	☐	☐

STATION 3.34

Examination

You are a medical student attached to the breast clinic. You are required to examine the breasts of a 35-year-old woman who complains of painful and lumpy breasts.

(5 minute station)

STATION 3.35

Investigation

A 61-year-old woman, diagnosed with a recurrent carcinoma of her right breast, underwent the staging investigations shown (fig 3.35a and 3.35b).

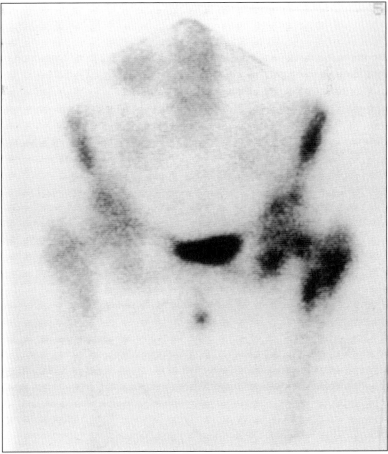

fig 3.35a

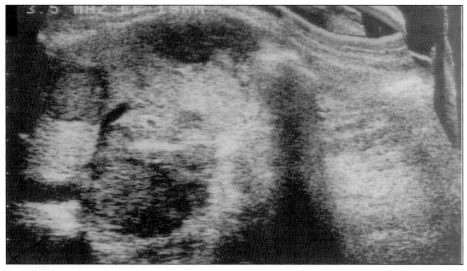

fig 3.35b

1 Please name the imaging procedures in fig 3.35a and 3.35b and describe the
   salient features in each.
2 State your conclusions from what you have observed.
3 Comment on how these findings influence the treatment of the primary breast
   lesion.

(5 minute station)

STATION 3.36

Investigation

Figs 1.34a and b are radiological examinations of the right breast in two middle-aged women taken during a community screening programme.

(5 minute station)

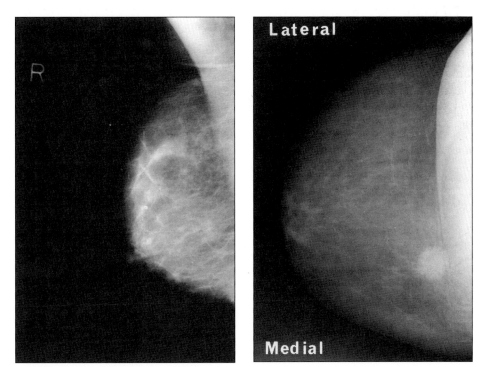

fig 3.36a   fig 3.36b

1 What are the radiographs called?

2 Indicate the abnormal findings in any one radiograph.

3 State your radiological diagnosis in each.

4 What other investigation would you perform to confirm the diagnosis?

5 How would you counsel these patients on the need for further assessment?

STATION 3.37

Investigation

Please perform a fine needle aspiration (FNA) for cytological examination of a breast lump marked on a plastic model.

(5 minute station)

Female manikin, syringe and fine needle, microscope slides, plain specimen bottle containing fixative, spray fixative for slides, sterile wipes, small adhesive dressing.

STATION 3.38

Treatment

A 40-year-old woman and her partner await the results of the triple assessment of a breast lump which was found to be malignant. Inform the patient (and partner) of the diagnosis and offer counselling.

(5 minute station)

Chapter 4:
Ethics and Legal Medicine, including Consent and IV Procedures

Contents

Chapter 4

Ethics and Legal Medicine, including Consent and IV Procedures

Ethics and legal issues – Introduction

Ethical and legal situations and dilemmas are faced by clinicians almost every working day. Such issues often pose difficulties to the medical student or junior doctor and are, therefore, avoided. Observation of senior colleagues and acquired experience help: the following simple guidelines may make dealing with these issues a little easier.

Ethical issues are often multifaceted. Difficult emotional and interpersonal dynamics direct the various parties involved in desiring different results. As doctors, one of the most difficult areas to confront is the lack of a definitive, correct answer. Such issues are often grey, and it is this uncertainty which troubles us all.

When dealing with these issues ask yourself whether the following items have been considered and answered.

- **'Do no harm'.** This simple principle should underpin everything one does in medicine. Within this phrase lies the issue of the 'patient's best interests'. At all times the patient is the one we are all working to help, and this may need to be impressed upon relatives and other healthcare professionals.

Doing no harm should also be applied to dealings with relatives and other healthcare professionals. Their views should be noted empathetically. It may be you who are 'wrong'! Doctors are often very poor at looking after themselves and one another. Doing no harm should also be applied to oneself and one's colleagues. Support for each other and yourself is very important. Medicine is a team game!

- **Communication**. It is always important to ensure careful documentation of discussions with colleagues, relatives and patients. Procedures and actions should be truthfully described, including mishaps and poor outcomes. This is not only a legal obligation and sensible professional practice, but it also allows colleagues to follow the rationale and direction of treatment.

- **Legal aspects.** Junior doctors are often unaware of the legal aspects and implications of their actions. In difficult situations it is always wise to seek a wide range of opinion from nursing staff, colleagues and other healthcare professionals involved with the case. Senior colleagues' advice, particularly that of the lead clinician, should be sought and noted. In very difficult or awkward situations the advice of the GMC, BMA, MDU or MPS should also be sought and noted.

- **Work towards compromise.** Within the framework set out above one must work towards compromise. The setting of realistic, achievable goals, and recognition of success and results should be acknowledged. Compromise between the interested parties may often be the only way to succeed in such matters.

STATION 4.1

You are the medical SHO on call. The House Officer has rung you to tell you that a 53-year-old woman in the Emergency Department is refusing treatment after being admitted with a paracetamol overdose.

On questioning the House Officer, you find out that she has serious suicidal intent but appears well orientated and rational. She has no psychotic symptoms.

Unfortunately, you are dealing with an emergency on one of the wards and cannot see the woman yourself. Please advise the House Officer how to proceed, protecting all the parties involved.

(10 minute station)

STATION 4.2

Preparatory
You have 5 minutes to read the information below before attempting the next station.

You are a GP in a large practice. One of your partners has left you a rather difficult situation to deal with. He has been seeing a 56-year-old woman, who had a genetic screening test for Huntington's chorea. She found out that her father committed suicide aged 50 when he was diagnosed as having the disorder. Her mother died when she was young, and neither her three brothers nor her two daughters know about their father's/grandfather's problem.

The test indicates that she has the disorder, but when your partner told her she refused to allow him to tell or screen her relatives. One of her daughters is your patient and is 'trying for a family'.

Please counsel the patient with a view to obtaining her consent to use this information to screen her family. Huntington's chorea is an autosomal dominant disorder, which causes progressive dementia and unwanted, involuntary movements. It is usually fatal.

(5 minute station)

STATION 4.2a

The 56-year-old woman, who is a patient of one of your partners, has come to see you for the results of her genetic screening test, which are positive for Huntington's chorea. Please counsel her with a view to obtaining her consent to use the information to screen her family.

(10 minute station)

STATION 4.3

Preparatory

You have 5 minutes to read the information below before attempting the next station.

You are a House Officer attending a care-planning meeting for a 79-year-old man with mild dementia. The gentleman has insisted on going home, but relatives, his primary carers, are refusing, as they say he is unsafe and is a danger to himself and his neighbours.

The salient points from the case notes are as follows:

On admission – found by police, very confused and wandering naked in the street.

Mental test score – 1/10.

Diagnosis – UTI/confusional state.

UTI treated with good effect, using oral trimethoprim.

Mental test score now 7–8/10

Rehabilitation: nurse's report – independent of all ADLs, very pleasant on the ward, a little slow mobilising.

Occupational therapist's report: home visit very successful, needs a few minor adjustments (ie handrail on the stairs and in the bathroom).

Physiotherapist's report: walks independently with a stick; a little slow sometimes. Occasionally unsteady but continues to improve.

Social worker's report: the patient has accepted that the gas must be capped off and meals on wheels brought in. Home care to help with cleaning; bath attendant arranged for once a week.

(5 minute station)

STATION 4.3a

You have been asked to present the case to the relatives as to why this 79-year-old gentleman with mild dementia is safe to go home.

This station may be acted out as a group OSCE, with people playing the roles of each member of the healthcare team (ie social worker, occupational therapists and physiotherapists and nurse).

(10 minute station)

STATION 4.4

Preparatory

You have 5 minutes to read the information below prior to attempting the next station.

You are the ITU consultant in a district general hospital. You have been called at home by your registrar for some advice. This is the dilemma that faces you both:

Case 1: In the last 5 minutes, an 83-year-old man has been admitted to the Emergency Department. He was riding his new mountain bike to see a friend when he was hit by a hit-and-run driver. He has multiple fractures and a head injury, and was electively paralysed and ventilated at the scene by the trauma team.

There are three beds in your ITU, and all are occupied.

Bed 1: A 68-year-old, previously fit and well woman, who, while recovering from a total hip replacement, developed a severe lower-respiratory tract infection, leading to acute respiratory distless syndrome (ARDS). She was electively ventilated 2 days ago and is stable. She is the mother of the Care of the Elderly physician.

Bed 2: A 24-year-old human immunodeficiency virus HIV-positive man, has systemic candidiasis, with cerebral involvement. During the last 24 hours he has required triple inotrope support and has worsening renal and cardiorespiratory function.

Bed 3: A 54-year-old businessman and leading local councillor, who was electively ventilated for respiratory distress, secondary to pulmonary oedema following an anterior myocardial infact (MI).

(5 minute station)

STATION 4.4a

As the ITU consultant you have to decide the most appropriate management for the four patients described in Station 4.4. Please discuss the factors that you take into account when deciding which patient to transfer to another hospital 20 miles away.

(10 minute station)

STATION 4.5

Counselling

A 30-year-old man is being treated by you, his general practitioner, for tonic-clonic seizures. His wife has informed you that, contrary to your advice not to drive, he continues to drive a minicab. You have asked to see the patient to discuss the situation. Please counsel the patient, with a view to reaching an agreement about his driving.

(10 minute station)

Informed consent

Informed consent may be written or verbal. It implies that the patient agrees to the procedure to which he or she is about to be exposed which is fully explained and any anxieties addressed.

In recent years, the medico-legal implications of poor consent have become much more prominent. House officers, who often have little knowledge or experience of technically complex procedures, have traditionally been the people required to obtain informed consent. This situation is unsatisfactory for patient, doctor and lawyer.

In recognition of these facts, the Royal Colleges have issued new guidelines which recommend that the person(s) performing the procedure should be the one(s) to obtain the informed consent.

The following stations represent common procedures that, although not directly performed in most instances by the junior doctor, are still procedures which one should be familiar with and obtain informed consent.

Important aspects of informed consent

How much information? The simple answer to this difficult question is as much as is necessary to impart all the information regarding the procedure, while answering all the patients' anxieties.

Students and newly-qualified/inexperienced doctors often avoid important and difficult parts of this process, as they find discussion awkward. Medico-legally this is disastrous. Experience and knowledge have made this a lot easier and although never easy, have led to the new guidelines.

Mortality and morbidity must be clearly explained and noted.

Who gives consent? If at all possible, the patient must be the one to give informed consent. Under common law, procedures may be undertaken in emergencies with the consent of two doctors. In patients less than 16 years old, a parent or guardian must give their consent. In all cases, the patient's wishes must always be respected, and patient confidentiality must be assured and maintained.

STATION 4.6

Informed consent: Preparatory
Please read the information below before attempting the next station.

(5 minute station)

You are the House Officer on a gastroenterology firm. You have been asked to obtain informed consent from a 52-year-old woman who has been admitted for a liver biopsy to be performed by your registrar this morning.

On review of the notes you ascertain the following facts:

    (a) Alcohol consumption – 5–10 units a day.

    (b) No risk factors for hepatitis B or C.

    (c) The consultant has diagnosed possible haemochromatosis.

    (d) The patient has already been clerked in pre-admission clinic.

No results of FBC or INR.

Common side-effects of the procedure:

    (a) Local bruising.

    (b) Right upper quadrant pain – mild to moderate.

    (c) Referred pain to the right shoulder.

OSCE Stations

Uncommon side-effects:

> (a) More severe abdominal pain as a result of bleeding from the liver.
> (b) Biliary peritonitis.
> (c) Haemobilia.

These may require admission and possible surgery.

Procedure
Takes 5 to 10 minutes

Patient reclines and takes a deep breath and holds it for 10 seconds

Needle passed into the liver and a small piece taken away

Procedure performed under local anaesthetic

Post-procedure
Must recline for 6 to 8 hours

Can go home after this period if observations are normal

Will have blood pressure/pulse taken half- to one-hourly through this period

NOTE: This procedure cannot be undertaken until an INR and platelet count are known.

STATION 4.6a

Informed consent
Please obtain informed consent from the 52-year-old woman who has been admitted for a liver biopsy to be performed by your registrar this morning.

(10 minute station)

STATION 4.7

Informed consent: Preparatory
Please read the following information before attempting the next station.

(5 minute station)

You are the medical House Officer attached to a gastroenterology firm. The next patient is a 43-year-old woman, who has been admitted to day care for an upper GI endoscopy. She was found to have a hypochromic microcytic anaemia on routine investigation.

Upper GI endoscopy – OGD = oesophagogastroduodenoscopy

Procedure
Performed under local anaesthetic which is sprayed at the back of the throat; occasionally the patient is given an intravenous sedative.

Endoscope is about 1 cm in diameter and is passed down through the gullet into the stomach.

It also allows biopsies to be taken.

Side-effects:

>   Common: sore throat and gullet, drowsiness if sedation used

>   Uncommon: Oesophageal tears – small, spontaneously heal; large

>   – pneumomediastinum, mediastinitis – requires antibiotics.

Larger tears may require surgery.

STATION 4.7a

Informed consent
You have been asked to obtain informed consent from this 43-year-old woman, who is being investigated for a microcytic anaemia for an upper GI endoscopy.

(5 minute station)

STATION 4.8

Informed consent: Preparatory
Please read the following information before attempting the next station.

(5 minute station)

You are a surgical House Officer, and you have been asked to obtain informed consent for a colonoscopy from a 62-year-old woman who is being investigated for weight loss and intermittent constipation.

Procedure:

Performed using intravenous sedation, which also has amnesic effect.

Endoscope is about 1 cm in diameter and is passed up through the anus.

The endoscope is flexible and carries a fibre-optic light which allows the inside of the bowel to be seen.

It also allows biopsies to be taken.

Side-effects:

Common: Discomfort during the procedure, bleeding from bowel lining.

Uncommon: Perforation of the bowel; small – treated conservatively with antibiotics; large – may need oversewing if detected early.

A defunctioning colostomy may be required if there is peritoneal soilage.

STATION 4.8a

Informed consent
You are required to obtain informed consent for a colonoscopy from this 62-year-old woman who is being investigated for weight loss and constipation.

(5 minute station)

STATION 4.9

Informed consent: Preparatory
Please read the following information before attempting the next station.

(5 minute station)

You are a House Officer attached to a gastroenterology firm. You have been asked to obtain informed consent for an ERCP from a 36-year-old obese woman. She presented 2 days ago with jaundice, and ultrasound has shown gallstones and a dilated common bile duct.

ERCP = endoscopic retrograde cholangiopancreatography

Procedure

Performed with a local anaesthetic spray in back of the throat and intravenous sedation.

Endoscope is flexible and carries a fibre-optic light, allowing the operator to view inside the bowel.

Need to identify and cannulate the ampulla of Vater so that a wire basket 'cage' will be passed up around stone and the operator will attempt to remove it. A small cut may be made in the sphincter of Oddi for this purpose. If unsuccessful, may require further attempt or operation.

Side-effects:

Common: sore throat and gullet

Uncommon: pancreatitis, cholangitis

OSCE Stations

STATION 4.9a

Informed consent
You are required to obtain informed consent for an ERCP from an obese 36-year-old woman who presented with jaundice secondary to a gallstone in the common bile duct. Please obtain informed consent and address any anxieties the patient may have.

(5 minute station)

STATION 4.10

Informed consent: Preparatory

Please read the information below. You have 5 minutes to prepare for the following station

You are a House Officer attached to a cardiology firm. You have been asked to obtain informed consent for a transoesophageal echocardiogram from a 43-year-old in-patient who is suspected of having infective endocarditis.

You will need to mention the following information:

(a) The patient is required to be conscious for the procedure as he or she needs to assist the operator by swallowing and moving from time to time. Normally local anaesthetic spray is used to anaesthetise the back of the throat. Anxious patients can have a small injection which will make them sleepy and stops them from remembering the procedure.

(b) The instrument is about 3–4 cm in diameter at its thickest and the patient is asked to swallow it down into their oesophagus/gullet.

(c) The procedure takes about 10 minutes and should be no more than uncomfortable.

Common complications :

(a) During the procedure the patient will gag on the instrument but should NOT feel any pain.

(b) Post-procedure the patient is often left with a slight sore throat and oesophagus. This will pass in a few days.

Uncommon complications : these are extremely rare

(a) The instrument may tear the oesophagus, causing pneumomediastinum (air in the mediastinum). Small tears will spontaneously heal over; larger tears may require surgical intervention.

(b) Surgical emphysema (air within the soft tissues and below the skin).

(c) Mediastinitis – severe sepsis within the mediastinum rarely this may be fatal.

(5 minute station)

STATION 4.10a

Informed consent

Please obtain informed consent from this 43-year-old in-patient who is suspected of having infective endocardiditis for a transoesophageal echocardiogram.

(5 minute station)

STATION 4.11

Informed consent: Preparatory

You are a House Officer attached to a cardiology firm. The next patient is a 53-year-old man who has been admitted for day case cardiac catheterisation. You have been sent to obtain informed consent from the patient who has already been clerked in the pre-admissions clinic.

(5 minute station)

Please obtain informed consent mentioning the following information:

- The procedure is performed under local anaesthetic.
- An injection is given into the groin and a very thin tube is passed up to the heart.
- Contrast medium is then injected in through the tube. This is a special fluid which shows up under X-ray. A cine-film is taken as it passes through the blood vessels and the heart.

From this information we can tell what is causing the chest pain.

The patient must lie in bed after the procedure for 4–6 hours before being allowed home

Must ensure the patient:

- Can lie flat for 20 minutes
- Has no previous reactions to medications or contrast media.

Common complications:

- Flushing/warm feeling as the contrast medium is circulating
- Bruising at the puncture site in the groin.

Uncommon complications:

- Rupture of a coronary artery requiring immediate bypass surgery
- Arrhythmia requiring treatment
- Death – mortality is less than 1%
- Femoral false aneurysm – requiring surgery.

OSCE Stations

STATION 4.11a

Informed consent
You have been asked to obtain informed consent from this 53-year-old man who has been admitted for day case cardiac catheterisation.

(5 minute station)

Generic skills
The following four stations are common to all branches of medicine from general practice to psychiatry. A manikin arm should be available in all clinical skills centres. If you do not have access to such an arm you can still practise the stations, explaining how you would proceed.

STATION 4.12

For this station you will require a manikin arm, a tourniquet, vacutainer, needles, syringe, blood bottles and gloves.

You are the medical student attached to a GP practice. You have been asked by the GP to obtain a full blood count sample from a 43-year-old woman, who is attending the surgery for lethargy.

Please obtain a sample using the manikin arm, explaining your actions as you proceed.

(5 minute station)

STATION 4.13

For this station you will require a manikin arm, intravenous cannula, alcohol wipe, tourniquet, dressing for cannula, gloves, saline flush, syringe/needle.

You are the medical student attached to an obstetric and gynaecology firm. You have been requested to insert an intravenous cannula into a 23-year-old primagravida, who requires intravenous heparin for a suspected pulmonary embolism (PE). Using the manikin arm, insert the cannula, explaining your actions as you proceed.

(5 minute station)

STATION 4.14

For this station you will require a manikin arm with cannula in situ, a bag of intravenous fluid (you can use stickers to change the content), giving set, gloves and a drip stand.

You are the House Officer attached to a general medical firm. You have been asked by the senior House Officer to set up and site an intravenous drip for a 63-year-old woman, who was admitted 24 hours ago in a hyperglycaemic coma. The fluid chart is provided. Using the manikin arm, please set up and site the intravenous drip.

(5 minute station)

STATION 4.15

For this station you will require: a vial of antibiotic powder, gloves, appropriate mixing fluid, alcohol wipe, needles/syringes, a manikin arm with cannula in situ (the arm should have an identity bracelet), normal saline flush, appropriate prescription chart.

You are the medical student attached to a surgical firm. You have been requested by the House Officer to draw up and give a dose of antibiotic for a patient who is 24 hours post-cholecystectomy.

Using the manikin arm and the equipment provided, draw up and give the antibiotic, explaining your actions as you proceed.

(5 minute station)

OSCE Stations

Chapter 1:
Paediatrics Answers

Chapter 1

Paediatrics Answers

STATION 1.1

Cardiovascular examination

This station can either use a real baby or a manikin. If a manikin is used, do not score the first row or ausculation findings.

Assessment	Good	Adequate	Poor/not done
1 Appropriate introduction (full name and role)	☐	☐	☐
2 Candidate washes their hands using the alcohol handwash provided (no marks if candidate only expresses the need to wash if handwash is provided)	☐	☐	☐
3 Looks and comments on cyanosis, pallor, tachypnoea, scars.	☐	☐	☐
4 Looks and comments on dysmorphic features	☐	☐	☐
5 Feels brachial or femoral pulse, comments on character	☐	☐	☐
6 Comments on presence/absence of femoral pulse	☐	☐	☐
7 Listens to heart in four recognised positions and at the back	☐	☐	☐
8 Correctly identifies murmur if present	☐	☐	☐
9 Listens for pulmonary oedema	☐	☐	☐
10 Feels for liver edge	☐	☐	☐
11 Offers to measure blood pressure	☐	☐	☐
12 Offers to perform growth measurements	☐	☐	☐
13 Does examination in professional manner	☐	☐	☐

Comment

Paediatric cardiovascular examination should be straightforward. The keys are to see if the child is either cyanosed or in heart failure and if the child has a scar. If the child is blue, there is a problem getting blood into the lungs. Most likely, the child has Fallot's tetralogy. If the child is tachypnoeic and pink (and does not have respiratory disease), the child will be in heart failure and is likely to have a VSD or AVSD. Scars may be midline (implying a curative operation such as VSD closure or Fallot's repair) or subclavicular, suggesting a palliative systemic-pulmonary shunt or a coarctation resection.

An alternative presentation will be a child with a murmur who is neither blue nor tachypnoeic. This will either be an innocent or pathological murmur. Innocent ones do not radiate, are quiet and precordial and the child is otherwise well. Some alter with position. If it is not innocent, the position where it is loudest gives a clue as to the cause and also its character. Those loudest below the nipples are pansystolic (VSD, Fallot's, AVSD) and those above ejection systolic (PDA, AS, coarctation). In an examination, never forget the femorals, the blood pressure or the weight.

STATION 1.2

Respiratory examination

This station can use a patient with no respiratory signs, or one with longstanding illness, such as CF or asthma.

Assessment	Good	Adequate	Poor/not done
1 Appropriate introduction (full name and role)	☐	☐	☐
2 Candidate washes their hands using the alcohol handwash provided (no marks if candidate only expresses the need to wash if handwash is provided)	☐	☐	☐
3 Inspects for cyanosis, clubbing, scars	☐	☐	☐
4 Inspects for tachypnoea, recession, expansion	☐	☐	☐
5 Listens for crackles, wheeze, breath sounds	☐	☐	☐
6 Correctly identifies ausculation findings	☐	☐	☐
7 Feels for expansion, tracheal position	☐	☐	☐
8 Percussion (but must justify why)	☐	☐	☐
9 Feels pulse (but must say for paradoxus or bounding as with CO_2 retention)	☐	☐	☐
10 Measures peak flow and offers to measure weight	☐	☐	☐
11 Keeps patient comfortable and at ease	☐	☐	☐
12 Does examination in professional manner	☐	☐	☐

Comment

The key to all paediatric examination is good observation. From a distance look for tachypnoea, distress and hyperexpansion (seen best from the side) or asymmetrical expansion. Auscultation is usually best in babies if they are quiet, but in older children expansion, percussion should take place first. Always explain to the child and examiner what you are doing. Never forget the peak flow and weight. Also, if you are doing something, be prepared to say why (there is little point percussing or eliciting vocal fremitus in a child with equal and normal breath sounds).

Common conditions in OSCEs are CF, asthma, chronic lung disease (ex-prem) or possibly a baby recovering from bronchiolitis. In CF there will probably be a mixture of inspiratory crackles and expiratory wheeze (many have asthma too) and may be underweight. Those with chronic lung disease often have some degree of chest deformity and scars on their hands from repeated cannulation.

STATION 1.3

Abdominal examination

Assessment	Good	Adequate	Poor/not done
1 Appropriate introduction (full name and role)	☐	☐	☐
2 Candidate washes their hands using the alcohol handwash provided (no marks if candidate only expresses the need to wash if handwash is provided)	☐	☐	☐
3 Looks and comments on jaundice, anaemia, and amount of body fat	☐	☐	☐
4 Looks and comments on distension and presence of scars	☐	☐	☐
5 Feels for superficial tenderness and comments	☐	☐	☐
6 Feels competently for liver, spleen, kidneys, masses and constipation	☐	☐	☐
7 Listens to abdomen and percusses any mass	☐	☐	☐
8 Correctly identifies findings	☐	☐	☐
9 Offers to look in mouth and in perianal area	☐	☐	☐
10 Inspects groins	☐	☐	☐
11 Offers to look at penis and scrotum	☐	☐	☐
12 Offers to look at growth measurements	☐	☐	☐
13 Does examination in professional manner	☐	☐	☐

Comment

The abdominal examination is relatively easy to set up for an OSCE station, as there are many children with stable splenomegally, jaundice, nephrotic syndrome and constipation. As with the other systems to be examined, observation is the key. Here this means systemic signs – jaundice, anaemia and weight loss, and looking for abdominal distension, visible peristalsis and scars. Ensure that you look for inguinal and renal scars. A competent examination should always be directed towards the presenting complaint – in this case distension. Causes could be organomegaly, a mass, constipation or ascites. Students frequently forget to properly examine the groin, anus, penis and testes. You will not be required to do a paediatric rectal, but you should offer to look at the perianal area and genitalia.

Other openers for a paediatric abdominal examination are jaundice (look for other signs of liver involvement, measure liver span) and weight loss. (Also look at body fat, listen for a murmur and for signs of chest involvement in CF.)

STATION 1.4

Growth

This station can be run with a child of any age, but will work best over 4 years. For a baby, a manikin will be used. For a manikin, the first item is not used.

Assessment	Good	Adequate	Poor/not done
1 Appropriate introduction (full name and role)	☐	☐	☐
2 Candidate washes their hands using the alcohol handwash provided (no marks if candidate only expresses the need to wash if handwash is provided)	☐	☐	☐
3 Explains what about to do	☐	☐	☐
4 Measures head circumference (three attempts)	☐	☐	☐
5 Selects appropriate length/height device	☐	☐	☐
6 Uses correct technique for length/height	☐	☐	☐
7 Weighs correctly, ensuring properly undressed	☐	☐	☐
8 Obtains all measurements with small error	☐	☐	☐
9 Plots three measurements accurately	☐	☐	☐
10 Describes current and past measurements	☐	☐	☐
11 Provides differential diagnosis	☐	☐	☐
12 Does examination in professional manner	☐	☐	☐

Comment

Growth assessment in children should be very easy, but may be difficult to do accurately. The head circumference is the largest repeatable circumference between the occiput and forehead. Three attempts should be used. Height is used over 2 years old and supine length under 2 years old. The eyes and ears should be horizontal (or vertical if supine), the heels together and gentle traction should be put on the mastoid process (and feet if supine). Weight should be done with only underclothes and no nappy.

Plotting on the centile chart is done with weeks under 1 and months thereafter. If there is information that the child was born early, it is worthwhile for the first year to allow for this when plotting the measurements.

In a growth station you are most likely to get a normal child or a manikin. A child with a syndrome is a possibility (small, light, small head), or one with microcephaly alone, or perhaps a hormonal problem (short and fat). Another possibility is a child failing to thrive with a systemic disease (relatively light, but height and head circumference maintained). The growth chart here shows a small child with normal growth.

STATION 1.5

Examination of the Head

This station can use a real neonate or a model. If a model is used, do not score the first row.

Assessment	Good	Adequate	Poor/not done
1 Appropriate introduction (full name and role)	☐	☐	☐
2 Explains purpose of examination to parent	☐	☐	☐
3 Candidate washes their hands using the alcohol handwash provided (no marks if candidate only expresses the need to wash if handwash is provided)	☐	☐	☐
4 Inspects for overall shape of head	☐	☐	☐
5 Looks for facial dysmorphic syndrome and position of ears	☐	☐	☐
6 Feels sutures	☐	☐	☐
7 Feels for anterior, posterior and third fontanelle	☐	☐	☐
8 Checks for fusion of the sutures	☐	☐	☐
9 Measures head circumference	☐	☐	☐
10 Does examination in professional manner	☐	☐	☐

Comment

This is a basic part of the baby check and any examination of a baby. You are looking for craniosynostosis (asymmetric shape, fused sutures); syndromes that cause a small head (most chromosomal ones, often associated with a third fontanelle between the anterior and posterior one); hydrocephalus (large head, splayed sutures, 'sunsetting' eyes); and signs of raised intracranial pressure (splayed sutures, bulging fontanelle).

You will get asked when the sutures close (6 weeks), when the posterior and anterior fontanelle close (3 and 9 months on average, respectively). You may also have to comment on an asymmetric head and give it a name. There are only five that you would be expected to know: brachycephaly, which is the head shape associated with Down's, which is short in the A-P dimension; microcephaly, which is just small; plagiocephaly, which is rhomboid when viewed from above; and scaphocephaly, which is enlongated in the A-P dimension and short in the transverse dimension.

STATION 1.6

Dysmorphology examination
This station can be run with any major syndrome, but numerically there are far more with Down's and Turner's than any other. Beyond these you will not be expected to get a diagnosis, just to describe the features.

Assessment	Good	Adequate	Poor/not done
1 Appropriate introduction (full name and role)	☐	☐	☐
2 Explains purpose of examination	☐	☐	☐
3 Candidate washes their hands using the alcohol handwash provided (no marks if candidate only expresses the need to wash ifhandwash is provided)	☐	☐	☐
4 Looks at face, examining eyes, nose, ears, mouth	☐	☐	☐
5 Looks and palpates abdomen and justifies why	☐	☐	☐
6 Looks at head shape, feels fontanelles	☐	☐	☐
7 Looks at neck and arms	☐	☐	☐
8 Looks at hands for creases, shape and shape of fingers	☐	☐	☐
9 Looks at chest and listens to heart	☐	☐	☐
10 Examines feet	☐	☐	☐
11 Examines spine	☐	☐	☐
12 Offers to measure and weigh the child	☐	☐	☐
13 Does examination systematically and in a professional manner	☐	☐	☐

Comment

The key to a good dysmorphology examination is to have a system. Start with the face, looking individually at the eyes and the palpebral fissure, nasal bridge, philtrum, mouth, ears (shape and position) and cranium (anterior fontanelle, sutures and head size). Next look at the neck for webbing, the arms for a wide carrying angle and the hands for a single palmar crease and their shape. The fingers and knuckles are sometimes affected in syndromes. The chest is next, looking for widely spaced nipples or scars suggesting heart surgery and listening for a murmur. Look in the abdomen for scars (duodenal atresia in Down's) and feel for organomegaly that may point towards a storage or metabolic disorder. Look at the feet for a sandle gap. Lastly look at the back for spina bifida. Don't forget to weigh and measure the patient.

In terms of presenting such a patient, if it is obvious that they have Down's, say so and then demonstrate the features. If not, it is acceptable to go through the findings without reaching a diagnosis.

STATION 1.7

Neurology examination

Assessment	Good	Adequate	Poor/not done
1 Appropriate introduction (full name and role)	☐	☐	☐
2 Explains purpose of examination	☐	☐	☐
3 Candidate washes their hands using the alcohol handwash provided (no marks if candidate only expresses the need to wash if handwash is provided)	☐	☐	☐
4 Looks and comments on posture	☐	☐	☐
5 Briefly looks at child overall (blindness, syndrome, gastrostomy, failure to thrive)	☐	☐	☐
6 Asks child to take toy and comments on ability	☐	☐	☐
7 Feels tone of upper and lower limbs	☐	☐	☐
8 Examines power and reflexes competently	☐	☐	☐
9 Looks for contractures and scars from their release	☐	☐	☐
10 Assesses primitive reflexes (grasp, plantars)	☐	☐	☐
11 Asks child to walk and run if appropriate	☐	☐	☐

Comment

Neurology cases in paediatric OSCEs will almost always be children with cerebral palsy. Other possibilities include: spinal muscular atrophy (lower motor neurone weakness only) and Duchenne muscular dystrophy (boys only, predominantly proximal weakness, occasional pseudohypertrophy of calves).

The paediatric neurology examination is fairly similar to the adult format. As before, observation is key. From the end of the bed look for an upper motor neurone or a hypotonic posture. Look also for associated defects, such as blindness, failure to thrive and deafness. The rest of the examination identifies the type of defect (UMN/LMN), its location (mono-, di-, hemi- or quadriplegia) and the extent to which this is limiting function. Arm function can be assessed with toys or writhing and leg function by walking.

Hypertonia tends to develop over time after the insult that caused the cerebral palsy, and affected children are often hypotonic in infancy.

STATION 1.8

Developmental examination

Most children used for such a station will be developmentally normal. But a child with cerebral palsy or a syndrome can be used or one who is younger than advertised, creating the impression of developmental delay.

Assessment	Good	Adequate	Poor/not done
1 Appropriate introduction (full name and role)	☐	☐	☐
2 Explains purpose of examination	☐	☐	☐
3 Candidate washes their hands using the alcohol handwash provided (no marks if candidate only expresses the need to wash if handwash is provided)	☐	☐	☐
4 Observation of child with comment	☐	☐	☐
5 Offers child bricks and comments	☐	☐	☐
6 Comments on hearing and vocalisation	☐	☐	☐
7 Demonstrates lack of head lag, sitting posture, inability to stand, attempt at crawling	☐	☐	☐
8 Comments on social interaction of child	☐	☐	☐
9 Presents findings to examiner in organised manner	☐	☐	☐
10 Accurate with assessment of developmental age	☐	☐	☐
11 Does examination in professional manner	☐	☐	☐

Comment

Developmental examination has a reputation as one of the harder stations. It need not be. Examiners are looking for order and careful observation. Development is split into four scales or systems: gross motor, fine motor/vision, hearing/speech and social. You will need to know a few normal milestones in each scale.

The best approach is to start by observing the child from a distance and seeing what they are able to do in each scale. Then allow the child to take a silent toy from you and see what their hands do (type of grip, transfers, casting). Next assess if the child is able to turn to sounds, although a silent room and special rattles are needed to do it properly. Then check the gross motor system, starting with the child on its back, lifting into a sitting position by its shoulders to look for head lag. In the sitting position look at the curvature of the spine and check for sideways sitting reflexes. Then pull to stand and see if they can stand and with how much support. Lastly put prone and see if he or she will lift the head, chest or even crawl off. Socially you may notice a smile or stranger wariness.

The examiner may want you to comment or present the examination. Stick to the developmental systems and is the most advanced skill they have in each and how old this makes them developmentally. You can then say if the child is appropriate for age, globally delayed or asymmetrically delayed.

STATION 1.9

Skin examination

Picture	Diagnosis	Management plan
fig 1.9a	Chickenpox	Reassure – it will resolve spontaneously
fig 1.9b	Meningococcal sepsis	Intravenous antibiotics
fig 1.9c	Café au lait patch	Reassure – it is a birthmark
fig 1.9d	Molluscum contagiosum	Reassure – it will resolve spontaneously
fig 1.9e	(Mongolian) blue spot	Reassure – it is a birthmark

Comment

It is worthwhile scanning through a picture atlas of birthmarks in paediatrics as children are easy to find with birthmarks, some of which may be associated with syndromes. Also children with another problem may have a birthmark that you are asked to comment on. Common ones are the blue spot (typically on the buttocks in dark-skinned children), the capillary haemangioma (also known as the port wine stain), which is commonest in the nape of the neck, the cavernous haemangioma (strawberry mark) and café au lait patches, which, if numerous, point to neurofibromatosis and other syndromes.

There are three neurocutaneous conditions – neurofibromatosis, Sturge–Weber syndrome and tuberous sclerosis.

STATION 1.10

Examination of gait

Assessment	Good	Adequate	Poor/not done
1 Appropriate introduction (full name and role)	☐	☐	☐
2 Explains purpose of examination	☐	☐	☐
3 Candidate washes their hands using the alcohol handwash provided (no marks if candidate only expresses the need to wash if handwash is provided)	☐	☐	☐
4 Observation of child with comment on facies, signs of UMN posture	☐	☐	☐
5 Observation of gait walking away and towards	☐	☐	☐
6 Examines balance	☐	☐	☐
7 Asks and observes run	☐	☐	☐
8 Categorises gait correctly	☐	☐	☐
9 Examines leg muscle tone, reflexes	☐	☐	☐
10 Offers to measure leg lengths	☐	☐	☐
11 Does examination in professional manner	☐	☐	☐

Comment

Gait is a hard station, but fortunately in paediatrics it will almost always be a child with cerebral palsy, and just occasionally with a muscular or LMN weakness. As with most other examination stations, a systematic approach is needed. Ask the child to walk about 10 metres away and then return. Things to look for are scissoring gait (legs adducted), toe-walking and the arms in an UMN posture, all suggesting hypertonia, often found with cerebral palsy. Occasionally there may be a cerebellar or co-ordination problem that can be examined with heel toe-walking or balance with eyes closed.

Confirm your findings with a brief neurologic examination on the couch. Look for scars of tendon releases, for increased tone and reflexes.

STATION 1.11

Newborn examination

Assessment	Good	Adequate	Poor/not done
1 Appropriate introduction (full name and role)	☐	☐	☐
2 Explains purpose of examination	☐	☐	☐
3 Candidate washes hands using the alcohol handwash provided (no marks if candidate only expresses the need to wash if handwash is provided)	☐	☐	☐
4 Observation of baby with comment on colour, respiratory rate	☐	☐	☐
5 Looks at facies – comments on eyes, ears, mouth, nose	☐	☐	☐
6 Feels cranium, fontanelle and sutures	☐	☐	☐
7 Undresses baby, looks for signs of respiratory distress, tachypnoea	☐	☐	☐
8 Listens to chest and heart in an orderly fashion	☐	☐	☐
9 Feels for femorals	☐	☐	☐
10 Observes abdomen for distension, palpates for masses and organomegaly	☐	☐	☐
11 Looks and comments on umbilical stump	☐	☐	☐
12 Examines genitalia and that anus is patent	☐	☐	☐
13 Examines limbs, looking for extra digits and abnormal creases	☐	☐	☐
14 Turns prone and looks and feels for spinal anomaly	☐	☐	☐
15 Offers to examines hips with Barlow's and Ortolani's tests	☐	☐	☐
16 Offers to look for cataracts	☐	☐	☐

Answers

17 Checks grasp reflexes, offers to elicit
startle reflex ☐ ☐ ☐

18 Measures head circumference ☐ ☐ ☐

19 Does examination in professional manner ☐ ☐ ☐

Comment

There is quite a lot to a good neonatal examination, but preparing for it is essential –
not only might it come up in an OSCE, but it is the basis of most examination
stations in babies.

As with many other stations, order is the key. Most paediatricians start at the top
and work down to the genitalia. Then they turn the child prone and check the spine
and lastly check the hips. This has usually woken the baby up and allows fundoscopy.
Try to do the observation and auscultation before the baby is upset.

STATION 1.12

Patient history

I am a 23-year-old mother of three. The family is my son, Carl, 5, Jayne, 3 and Emmie, 9 months old. My partner and I have recently separated. All the family are well apart from Jayne, who has mild asthma (controlled with a blue puffer when needed) and me, as I also have asthma and frequent chest infections.

I am worried that Emmie is not growing properly and is a very picky eater. In my red book, the growth chart shows she is very small for her age. Emmie has a 6 oz bottle of milk when she wakes up, midmorning, at lunch time, teatime and just before bed. Although I offer her jars of food, toast, porridge she will not take more than a spoonful before turning her head away. The only solid food she will eat is chocolate and crisps.

She has been otherwise well. She was born at 35 weeks but left hospital after 10 days. There were no problems. She was found to have a heart murmur but this had gone at her 6-week check. There are no concerns about her development.

I have felt quite low recently, since my partner left and am getting frustrated by the children. Carl is very boisterous and runs around the flat. He often hits his sister. Emmie cries frequently and is difficult to settle. Sometimes I am tempted to hit her hard just to shut her up. I am feeling very isolated, and am not getting support from anyone – either friends, family or social services.

Assessment	Good	Adequate	Poor/not done
1 Appropriate introduction (full name and role)	☐	☐	☐
2 Establishes nature of problem	☐	☐	☐
3 Takes comprehensive failure to thrive history	☐	☐	☐
4 Establishes mother's isolation	☐	☐	☐
5 Takes adequate diet history	☐	☐	☐
6 Takes full family and social history	☐	☐	☐
7 Uncovers potential non-accidental injury	☐	☐	☐
8 Checks with mother information correct	☐	☐	☐

9 Takes history in empathic manner	☐	☐	☐
10 Makes reasonable management plan	☐	☐	☐
11 Does all in fluent and professional manner	☐	☐	☐

Diagnosis

Non-organic growth faltering. Unsupported and possibly depressed mother. Milk drinking baby.

Comment

A paediatric history station can be a challenge, but is fairly easy for examiners to create scenarios for actors that test communication skills and applied knowledge in a variety of specialites and acute and chronic settings. Fortunately, a considerable number of marks are always available for good practice and this means a proper introduction – full name, designation and purpose of interview. You need to ask open-ended questions, listen properly, be empathic and check the information you have received. If you are asked to summarise, only mention the key facts. There is often concern about the order of a paediatric history. The truth is that it does not matter much, as long as there is completeness and a flow to it. Start by looking properly into the presenting complaint, then ask most relevant questions – probably the PMH or FH, maybe the neonatal history. Tidy up loose ends at the finish, such as immunisation or development unless these are relevant to the presenting problem.

Failure to thrive is a common paediatric presentation. A non-organic cause is most likely, as with Emmie, who has a poor diet and stress at home. Coeliac disease, cystic fibrosis, cerebral palsy and VSDs are the commonest organic causes. A good history will ask about the diet, stools, infections, murmurs and development.

STATION 1.13

Patient history

I am Michelle, a 32-year-old mother. My only child is Maisie, who is 14 months old. She has had a cold for the last few days with a fever. The temperature has been up to 40°C, but I have been using Calpol to control the fever on the advice of my GP.

Today Maisie was having her lunchtime bottle when she looked a bit vacant, then went stiff. Her eyes went up into her head and she started shaking all over. I carried her out into the street still shaking and screamed for some help. The neighbour called for an ambulance. Before the ambulance came she had stopped – it probably lasted 5 minutes. Then she was asleep and unrousable. I did not notice her colour changing during the episode. After arrival in casualty she woke up and took some more Calpol as she was hot again. Now she wants to play again.

In the past she has been very well. She was born at term with no problems. She is fully immunised. She has just learnt to walk and is starting to say words. She can pick small objects up with her fingers. In the family, we are all well and there is no epilepsy, although my mother-in-law has mentioned that my husband had fits as a child.

Assessment	Good	Adequate	Poor/not done
1 Appropriate introduction (full name and role)	☐	☐	☐
2 Establishes nature of problem	☐	☐	☐
3 Takes comprehensive history of current illness	☐	☐	☐
4 Takes comprehensive history of the fit	☐	☐	☐
5 Takes full background history – development and PMH	☐	☐	☐
6 Takes family history	☐	☐	☐
7 Checks with mother is information correct	☐	☐	☐
8 Takes history in empathic manner	☐	☐	☐
9 Makes reasonable management plan	☐	☐	☐
10 Does all in fluent and professional manner	☐	☐	☐

Diagnosis

Probable febrile convulsion.

Comment

Assessment of a child with fits is another common history station. All the generic skills (see above) are still important. Here you have to be clear what you are trying to do with the history. The commonest cause of fits in children is febrile convulsions (2% of the population). This is, however, a diagnosis of exclusion – it might be a presentation of epilepsy, meningitis, encephalitis, a tumour, metabolic disorder or even related to cerebral palsy. Things to ask about are if the convulsion had a focal element, any impairment of consciousness before or after the fit, or if there is any developmental delay. If these features are not present and the child is in the febrile convulsion age (9 months to 3 years), most paediatricians manage these children by looking for the source of the fever and symptomatic treatment. If there are these other features, an EEG, CT or MRI would be needed.

STATION 1.14

Patient History

I am Laura, Alfie's mother. He is 6 months old and he has a 4-year-old sister, Rosie. For the last week he has had a runny nose, mild fever and cough. Over the last few days his cough has got much worse and seems to come in bouts, during which he finds it difficult to catch his breath. It seems to be a chesty cough. His sister too has had a cough for the last few weeks, but I think this is her asthma. Alfie's cough is perhaps a bit worse during the daytime, although it does wake him up. Sometimes the cough is so bad he vomits afterwards and he went blue with it earlier this evening. That was the reason I brought him in now. He was seen 2 days ago by the GP who thought that he had a virus and did not prescribe any antibiotics.

Alfie has been very well up to now. He is up to date with his immunisations except pertussis, which I excluded as it can cause a reaction. He is starting to crawl and babble and uses his hands well. His growth has been normal, and his birth was painful and slow but without medical problems.

Assessment	Good	Adequate	Poor/not done
1 Appropriate introduction (full name and role)	☐	☐	☐
2 Establishes nature of problem	☐	☐	☐
3 Takes comprehensive history of current illness	☐	☐	☐
4 Takes comprehensive history of coughing spells – includes vomiting and cyanosis	☐	☐	☐
5 Takes full background history – development, PMH and immunisations	☐	☐	☐
6 Takes family history	☐	☐	☐
7 Checks with mother information correct	☐	☐	☐
8 Takes history in empathic manner	☐	☐	☐
9 Makes reasonable management plan	☐	☐	☐
10 Does all in fluent and professional manner	☐	☐	☐

Diagnosis

Whooping cough in an unimmunised child.

Comment

This history station illustrates why a full family and immunisation history is crucial. Here the other possibilities are asthma (a bit too young), bronchiolitis (a bit too old), croup (wrong cough), chest infection (not that septic) and an upper respiratory-tract infection (cough too bad). Pertussis is fairly common because of poor immunisation coverage and waning immunity. If school-age children are affected, there is a persistent cough that is no more than annoying. The younger the child is, the more serious it can be, with the very young having apnoeas, hypoxic spells and even neurological consequences. It causes a lymphocytosis and can be diagnosed with a per-nasal swab. It can be treated with erythromycin if given in the first 7 days.

STATION 1.15

Patient history

I am Jane, the mother of Rory, who is 9 months old. He has been well for the last few months. He was born at 29 weeks and was ventilated for 2 weeks. He had an episode of suspected necrotising enterocolitis, but this settled with antibiotics. He came off oxygen at 6 weeks of age and since then has done well. He has always been small for his age, even when his prematurity is taken into account. His recent follow-up appointments have been very positive – the doctors are pleased with his progress and his development.

This episode started yesterday. He seemed not to be hungry, even for his milk and in the evening he was sick. He was sick several times after that, at first, 'milk with lumps in and now greenish water'. At first I thought it was gastroenteritis, but there has been no diarrhoea. Instead his tummy has blown up a little and at times he seems in pain with this, pulling up his knees. Half an hour ago he opened his bowels, but all he passed was a bit of bloody mucus. My partner is well and there are no other people in the family. All the rest of us are well.

Assessment	Good	Adequate	Poor/not done
1 Appropriate introduction (full name and role)	☐	☐	☐
2 Establishes nature of problem	☐	☐	☐
3 Takes comprehensive history of current illness	☐	☐	☐
4 Takes comprehensive history of the neonatal period	☐	☐	☐
5 Takes full background history – development and PMH	☐	☐	☐
6 Checks correct information with mother	☐	☐	☐
7 Takes history in empathic manner	☐	☐	☐
8 Makes reasonable management plan	☐	☐	☐
9 Does all in fluent and professional manner	☐	☐	☐

Diagnosis
Intussusception.

Comment
The causes of vomiting are many. Here there is an abdominal cause, but the child may also have appendicitis or an obstruction due to a congenital abnormality, a hernia, a volvulus or adhesions. Children will often vomit if they have a fever, or have a cough. Babies with gastro-oesophageal reflux or pyloric stenosis will also vomit. A good history can usually separate most of these causes.

You may be asked what you would look for on examination. As with the history, assess signs of systemic illness (shock, fever, dehydration, reduced consciousness level) and then signs that might suggest a diagnosis (distension, hernias, bowel sounds).

Investigations will also aim to assess the impact of the vomiting (U+Es) and look for a cause; also plain films, ultrasound or contrast enemas. Here, with a history suggestive of intussusception, an ultrasound could be used to make the diagnosis and an air enema to treat.

A station like this may leave you a bit stumped. If you have no idea what is going on, it is usually best to talk sense. You could say that the bilious vomiting and the distension point to obstruction, even if you do not know what the cause is.

STATION 1.16

1	(D)	(e)
2	(E)	(d)
3	(A)	(b)
4	(B)	(a)
5	(C)	(c)

Comment

With some OSCE questions you can prepare by lots of practise, but others require some knowledge. This is such a question. Here it is important to be very careful and look at all the information available.

Here you can start with the hypotensive child. Causes in a previously well child are meningococcus, pneumococcus and haemophilus, but only meningococcus produces a purpuric rash. Of the organisms in the table, only *Haemophilus* is a common cause of otitis media.

CNS infection is also caused by meningococcus, pneumococcus and haemophilus. Some viruses can cause encephalitis of which only two are notable – chickenpox, which can cause a cerebellar encephalits and herpes simplex, which can be very serious. UTIs in children are caused by bowel organisms, particularly *Eschelichia coli*. Chest infections are frequently viral, but bacterial infections can be caused by a wide variety of organism, including pneumococcus and mycoplasma.

STATION 1.17

1	(B)	(d)
2	(D)	(a)
3	(A)	(e)
4	(E)	(b)
5	(C)	(c)

Comment

This station again requires some knowledge, but is intended to mimic the clinical situation where you have to choose between a number of possibilities.

STATION 1.18

Neonatal Cardiopulmonary Resuscitation

Assessment	Good	Adequate	Poor/not done
1 Looks for signs of life	☐	☐	☐
2 Airway opening manoeuvre	☐	☐	☐
3 Applies bag and mask	☐	☐	☐
4 Inflates chest	☐	☐	☐
5 Checks for pulse	☐	☐	☐
6 Initiates CPR in correct place	☐	☐	☐
7 Correct rate/ratio of breaths/compression	☐	☐	☐
8 Reassesses clinical state	☐	☐	☐
9 Does all smoothly and calmly	☐	☐	☐

Comment

Neonatal CPR is a compulsory part of most medical courses. There are many books on the subject and you should prepare properly for neonatal, child and adult CPR, with and without equipment. It often crops up in OSCEs, as it is so easy to put on such a station. The key, beyond of course knowing what to do, is order, reassessment and looking calm.

The order is assessment of the situation, calling for help, airway, breathing, circulation and reassessment. For paediatrics there is the added challenge of age and size appropriate guidelines. Neonatal masks come in three sizes, with the middle one being the only one of any use for a term baby. There is a large range for older children. The principle is that it must cover the mouth and nose and not leak. Laerdel bag sizes are also age appropriate, with the 500 ml one being most used for neonates. If you are asked, a size 3.5 endotracheal tube is appropriate for a neonate.

Compressions should be one finger breadth below the internipple line (neonate) and the lower sternum at older ages. At all ages you can use 100/min, compressing a third the depth of the chest with a 1:5 ratio. You should be able to feel a femoral pulse and see the chest move with your measures.

STATION 1.19

Paediatric airway

Assessment	Good	Adequate	Poor/not done
1 Looks for signs of life	☐	☐	☐
2 Airway opening manoeuvre	☐	☐	☐
3 Applies bag and mask	☐	☐	☐
4 Inflates chest	☐	☐	☐
5 Checks for pulse	☐	☐	☐
6 Reassesses clinical state	☐	☐	☐
7 Discusses options	☐	☐	☐
8 Does all smoothly and calmly	☐	☐	☐

Comment

As with the previous station, you need to know this area as it will come up. Again ensure that you have the right-sized equipment and that you are constantly monitoring your resuscitation success – is the chest moving?

You may be asked at the end of basic life support procedure to comment on what next. This usually will involve more senior people, intubation and paediatric intensive care unit (PICU). Principles are vital to this – aim for stability in each system (ABC) under the headings 'equipment' and 'monitoring'. Airway – the best equipment is a secured endotracheal tube, its position checked on chest radiograph. Monitor airway by seeing the chest rise, pulse oximetry and blood gases. Breathing – for stability you need a ventilator, with settings appropriate to the child (you do not need to know these!) and monitor as for airway. Circulation – the equipment you need is two large bore cannulae or a central venous line. Fluid boluses or inotropes may be needed, and monitoring is with ECG, blood pressure and clinical signs such as capillary perfusion.

STATION 1.20

Respiratory explanation

Assessment	Good	Adequate	Poor/not done
1 Appropriate introduction (full name and role)	☐	☐	☐
2 Explains purpose of discussion	☐	☐	☐
3 Correctly assembles equipment	☐	☐	☐
4 Explains purpose of inhalers	☐	☐	☐
5 Demonstrates how to use	☐	☐	☐
6 Checks mother understands theory and when to use	☐	☐	☐
7 Checks and advises mother's technique	☐	☐	☐
8 Does above in supportive and non-critical manner	☐	☐	☐
9 Organised approach	☐	☐	☐

Comment

Explanation stations require an element of knowledge, but also incorporate lots of technique that can be learnt and practised. The essence of this technique is to find out what it known, to inform in a way appropriate to that knowledge, then to find out that the information has been understood. Always use language appropriate to the recipient. Package your information and questions into small chunks and concentrate on demonstration where possible. These principles are even more important if there is an interpreter.

Asthma and diabetes are typical settings for an explanation station. With asthma in children it is vital to get equipment age appropriate for the child and then to check they are being used properly. Many carers are concerned about using steroids and need reassurance. Mistakes include using the steroids before the B_2 agonist and not rinsing out the mouth after steroids.

Metered dose inhalers can only be used in teenagers. Dry powder inhalers such as the turbohaler work for the over 5s and you will have to use a spacer device for those under that age. For children under 2-years old you will probably need a mask fitted on to the end of the spacer because the child will not make a seal around the exit valve.

STATION 1.21

Respiratory explanation

Assessment	Good	Adequate	Poor/not done
1 Appropriate introduction (full name and role)	☐	☐	☐
2 Explains purpose of discussion to mother	☐	☐	☐
3 Engages child in discussion	☐	☐	☐
4 Puts device together and demonstrates	☐	☐	☐
5 Teaches child how to use, best of three techniques	☐	☐	☐
6 Explains what readings mean	☐	☐	☐
7 Outlines how to use readings in an asthma management plan	☐	☐	☐
8 Checks information understood, clarifying if need be	☐	☐	☐
9 Does above in supportive and non-critical manner	☐	☐	☐
10 Uses appropriate language	☐	☐	☐

Comment

This station uses many of the same generic communication skills examined in the previous station. Here we also have a child to communicate with. Doing this well is an art that takes years, but you can learn some basic techniques quickly – skills that you can use in history taking stations too.

Young children like to know that their parents are comfortable with the situation, so talk to the parent first and explain what will happen. Then address the child. Get on their level – physically and with your language. If you are explaining a technique, take it slowly. Use lots and lots of encouragement. Never ask a child 'Would you like to...?' or 'Can you...?'

Peak flow devices should be used as part of a management plan, so that the reading is used to adjust the amount of inhaler used.

STATION 1.22

Therapeutics

First name _____   **Second name** _____

Date of Birth ____-____-____   **Unit number** _____

Drug Name	Dose	Frequency	Days supply	Duration	Pharmacy

Prescriber's name _____ **Signature** _____ **Date** ____-____-____

---

fig 1.22b

Mark sheet for prescription form

Correct patient information

Selects trimethoprim

Chooses treatment dose 4 mg/kg bd as mg

Chooses prophylactic dose 2 mg/kg od as mg

Specifies treatment course length 2–10 days

Signs form

Comment
This station requires knowledge of how to treat a UTI, how to choose an antibiotic and prescribe for children.

As you can see from the score sheet there are easy marks to pick up just by filling out the form and signing it. From the selection of antibiotics in the sensitivity sheet you have to choose an oral antibiotic that is appropriate for a child of this age (only trimethoprim) and prescribe it at an appropriate weight dose. The last marks are for acting on the knowledge that antibiotics for a UTI need not only treat the UTI but then, at a lower dose, act as prophylaxis.

STATION 1.23

Explanation of results

I am Megan Young, mother of Mark. I have brought him to the hospital to find out the results of the tests carried out over the last 2 weeks at the hospital. There were some blood tests, a urine test and a test where Mark's sweat test was collected. I was told this was for cystic fibrosis, but this is unlikely because Mark has not had any breathing problem, and there is none in the family. I live with my partner and Mark is our first son.

Assessment	Good	Adequate	Poor/not done
1 Appropriate introduction (full name and role)	☐	☐	☐
2 Explains purpose of discussion to mother	☐	☐	☐
3 Checks understanding of purpose of investigations	☐	☐	☐
4 Explains result suggestive, but not conclusive for CF	☐	☐	☐
5 Explains why result not conclusive	☐	☐	☐
6 Outlines plan for further investigation (another sweat test, stool fat, genetics)	☐	☐	☐
7 Checks information understood, clarifying if need be, offering to write down	☐	☐	☐
8 Does above in supportive manner	☐	☐	☐
9 Uses appropriate language	☐	☐	☐

Comment

Explaining a result to a parent is another special communication skill. Although the temptation is to get to the point of the interview, you must first find out how much the parents already know, so that you can build on this information with the test result. You will often be asked to break bad news, as here. A slow, stepwise approach to the interview is therefore best, delivering appropriate information in 'chunks', checking that each is received before moving on to the next bit.

In this situation, the test is non-diagnostic, as there is insufficient sweat, a common problem in infants. It will have to be repeated, or a diagnosis made with genetics.

STATION 1.24

Explanation

I am Laura Westlake, a 35-year-old first time mother. Florence is 3 months old and has been born by caesarean section (she was breech) after an uneventful pregnancy. I have stopped work as a solicitor while Florence is young. Florence has been very well apart from the few days after the first set of vaccines, when she developed a fever of 37.9+°C and was a little bit unsettled. This settled on its own. I thought about giving her Calpol, but did not want to use drugs for such a young baby. After the vaccines she was left with a lump in her leg where one of the vaccine went in. The rest of my family are all very healthy, and neither my husband nor I can remember any problems with vaccines.

Assessment	Good	Adequate	Poor/not done
1 Appropriate introduction (full name and role)	☐	☐	☐
2 Elicits mother's concerns	☐	☐	☐
3 Empathic to mother	☐	☐	☐
4 Gives accurate and appropriate information on the vaccination	☐	☐	☐
5 Discusses benefits and drawbacks of vaccination	☐	☐	☐
6 Suggests helpful action	☐	☐	☐
7 Summarises and concludes interview	☐	☐	☐
8 Does not dismiss mother's concerns	☐	☐	☐
9 Overall handling of situation	☐	☐	☐

Comment

Vaccination comes up in many different places in medical exams, and any candidate would be wise to know immunisation schedules and the common vaccine side-effects and the contraindications. Here the mother is describing the normal reaction to the DPT vaccine, which often causes a mild fever and a little irritability, and is easily controlled with paracetamol. The lump is a common result of the HIB vaccine and goes in a few months. MMR will often cause fever, rash or facial swelling 1 week after the vaccine. Such stations will be assessed on how you use communication skills with appropriate knowledge. The steps involved in doing it well are summarised in the mark scheme in fig 1.24b.

STATION 1.25

Paediatric explanation – asthma

I am Clare, mother of Connor, aged 3 and Elaine, age 1. They, and my husband Gary, are well apart from the eczema Elaine and I have.

The asthma attack that Connor had came right out of the blue – he had no problems before apart from a tickly cough at night. He suddenly became very ill with difficulty catching his breath, but responded promptly to the nebulisers at the hospital. Now he is back to normal, although his night-time cough is a little worse. He takes the inhaler that was given to him at the hospital but it is a struggle. I would like to take him off the inhaler but am not sure this is the right thing to do. Both Gary and I smoke. We have no pets.

Assessment	Good	Adequate	Poor/not done
1 Appropriate introduction (full name and role)	☐	☐	☐
2 Confirms information in letter	☐	☐	☐
3 Finds out about Connor's current state	☐	☐	☐
4 Elicits mother's concerns	☐	☐	☐
5 Empathic to mother	☐	☐	☐
6 Discusses increasing treatment	☐	☐	☐
7 Summarises and concludes interview	☐	☐	☐
8 Does not dismiss mother's concerns	☐	☐	☐
9 Overall handling of situation	☐	☐	☐

Comment

This explanation station is a little different. You are asked to review treatment after a hospital discharge, but things are not going well. Connor still has symptoms of ongoing airways inflammation – the nocturnal cough. The best management for this situation is to introduce a regular inhaled steroid and discuss stopping smoking. However, the mother has a different agenda. Handling this well will require you to listen carefully to what she has to say, and then explain, without belittling her, that another plan is needed.

STATION 1.26

Investigation – chest radiograph

Comment

You will not be expected to go far beyond simple chest radiograph appearances in paediatrics and neonates, although you may encounter some very obvious radiographic findings in other systems. For example, rickets or non-accidental injury may be seen in limb radiographs and really dramatic obstruction, perforation, NEC or constipation in an abdominal film. You might also be expected to comment on a micturating cystourethrogram or isotope renal scan. Most radiology questions focus on the chest, where there will be neonatal, cardiovascular and respiratory films. In the neonate, RDS, diaphragmatic hernia and meconium aspiration are possible. The cardiovascular films either show a globular heart and pulmonary oedema, or a boot-shaped heart and oligaemic lung fields. The respiratory films show collapse, consolidation, hyperexpansion (asthma and bronchiolitis) or a pneumothorax.

Examiners first want to see that you know the anatomy and that you have a system for looking at the film. Reaching a diagnosis is good too!

This is the correctly competed table:

    (a)   Endotracheal tube

    (b)   Stomach bubble

    (c)   Umbilical arterial catheter

    (d)   Right main bronchus

    (e)   Lung field – demonstrates groundglass appearance

STATION 1.27

Paediatric investigations

1 Identifies enlarged heart.
2 Identifies plethoric lung fields.
3 Has system for reporting radiograph.
4 Suggests reasonable differential diagnosis.
5 Suggests investigation plan.
6 Suggests diuretics and diet.

Comment

System is the key to most data interpretation stations. Start with the bones, looking for fractures and evidence of rickets, then move to the soft tissues. Most babies are a little bit fat, so minimal soft tissue under the arms suggests long-term illness or malnutrition, especially cystic fibrosis. Next look at the heart, for size (the chest radiograph should be under 0.5) and shape. The shapes you will see are normal, globular (heart failure, effusion) or right ventricle dominant (Fallot's, pulmonary atresia). Then look at the abdomen, checking the stomach bubble is in the right place and there is no evidence of perforation. Lastly look at the lung fields. Assess them for hyperexpansion (flat diaphragms, thin heart, more than five and a half anterior rib ends seen). Look for oligaemia or plethora. Look at any opacity, describing its distribution and its nature. It will either be fluid tumour, or in a child, consolidation or collapse. These last two can be distinguished by air bronchograms and lack of volume loss in consolidation. Many paediatric respiratory problems are complicated by mucus plugging, leading to collapse.

Using this system it is obvious that there is an enlarged heart and the lung fields are opacified, particularly the upper zones. The pattern is non-lobar and bilateral. Although such a pattern may be found with some atypical chest infections, this is unlikely to also cause cardiomegaly. The most correct response in such a station is that the appearances are the result of pulmonary oedema of cardiac cause.

Management will involve investigations – an echocardiogram, ECG and urea and electrolytes to identify the cause and look for any renal effect. Management will involve diuretics and diet. Depending on the cause, surgery may be needed.

STATION 1.28

Paediatric investigations

This investigation is a micturating cystourethrogram (MCUG). It shows severe (grade 4) vesico-ureteric reflux. If the candidate does not realise what the investigation is, you may tell the candidate, and then ask what it shows. Once the candidate has described the reflux ask what this means anatomically. Then ask what this means for the child, who will need continued prophylactic antibiotics or even surgery.

1 Correctly identifies as MCUG.
2 Explains process of performing MCUG.
3 Explains findings on investigation anatomically, ie vesico-ureteric reflux.
4 Identifies reflux as severe.
5 Outlines future management plan.
6 Does all in competent and fluent manner.

Comment

As with interpretation of other investigations in an OSCE, an orderly approach is vital. The first problem is correctly identifying the test. The investigations used in the assessment of UTIs are DMSA, DTPA and MAG3 – all isotope scans; the MCUG, which looks at retrograde flow from the bladder to the ureters; the renal ultrasound, which screens for renal scars and gross ureteric dilation. The IVU is rarely used, but is useful if there is ureteric obstruction. This differs from the MCUG in that the renal cortex can also be seen.

Any degree of reflux is abnormal. Most reflux improves with time, but while present predisposes to UTIs, which may cause renal scarring. Hence children with reflux are treated with prophylactic antibiotics.

STATION 1.29

Paediatric ECG

Instructions for examiner:
Ask the candidate to report the ECG. It shows third-degree heart block with normal P wave and QRS axis for a neonate (ie right axis deviated, with a large QRS complex in the right chest leads). Ask the candidate what should be checked in the mother, and what you would assess in the baby.

If there is time, ask the candidate how the baby should be managed.

Assessment	Good	Adequate	Poor/not done
1 Comments on ventricular bradycardia	☐	☐	☐
2 Comments on third-degree heart block	☐	☐	☐
3 Has system to report ECG	☐	☐	☐
4 Correctly identifies right deviated axis	☐	☐	☐
5 Mentions SLE or anti-ro/anti-la antibodies	☐	☐	☐
6 Describes examination looking for heart failure in an infant	☐	☐	☐
7 Mentions diuretics, pacing	☐	☐	☐

Comment
The paediatric ECG is much less useful than the adult ECG as most paediatric heart conditions are structural, with normal muscle arranged abnormally rather than diseased muscle giving rise to rhythm disorders. If you are shown a paediatric ECG, it will either be a heart block and SVT, or a conduction disorder in a child with congenital heart disease.

Heart block in an otherwise normal heart is usually complete and congenital. Maternal SLE is the usual cause. Pacing is usually required, as the ventricular escape rate is too low to maintain adequate cardiac output. Look for signs of heart failure (respiratory difficulty arising from pulmonary oedema, hepatomegally, poor weight gain). SVT may present with similar signs, but usually does not become symptomatic until the HR is over 200.

The key to any ECG station is system. Look at rhythm, then P wave size and axis, then PR interval, then the QRS shape, and if there is no evidence of conduction block, the axis and the T waves. Neonates are very right axis deviated, with large QRS complexes and inverted T waves in V1 to V3, so technicians put the leads on the right of the chest, these are called V4R or RV4.

STATION 1.30

Paediatric radiology and management

Instructions for the examiner:
Ask the candidate for a report on the chest radiograph. Ask the candidate to identify the cause of the right upper lobe opacity. Then ask the candidate for a differential diagnosis. Lastly ask for a management plan.

Assessment	Good	Adequate	Poor/not done
1 Comments on RUL opacity	☐	☐	☐
2 Comments of hyperexpansion	☐	☐	☐
3 Has complete system to report radiograph	☐	☐	☐
4 Identifies collapse in RUL	☐	☐	☐
5 Differential succinct and accurate	☐	☐	☐
6 Management plan covers diagnosis and specific treatment	☐	☐	☐
7 Management plan provides supportive care for baby	☐	☐	☐

Comment

Again a system is vital to do well in a radiology station. Use the system described in question 1.27. This child is very likely to have bronchiolitis, with collapse and hyperexpansion. He is too young for asthma, although similar findings may be seen there. Chest infection, either viral or bacterial is possible, but there is little to see apart from collapse, which is not necessarily caused by chest infection.

A good plan would be diagnosis (nasopharyngeal aspirate, blood culture and infection markers). Depending on this the child could be put on an antibiotic. He will also need supportive care – oxygen, fluids or nasogastic feeds.

Chapter 2:
Obstetrics and
Gynaecology Answers

Chapter 2
Obstetrics and Gynaecology Answers

STATION 2.1

Patient History

I have been married for 3 years and I work full-time as an administrative officer for a pharmaceutical company. My husband is a civil engineer with a road construction firm. I had a miscarriage at 8 weeks 2 years ago and was admitted as an emergency and required an 'evacuation of the womb'. I have had no other pregnancies.

I was on the combined oral contraceptive pill until 6 months ago, when we decided to start a family. My last period was 10 weeks ago and they have always been 28 days, regular and of normal duration. My last cervical smear was 1 year ago and was normal (as they have all been). I have been feeling sick most mornings, have marked breast tenderness and am passing urine more frequently than normal. I do not smoke but drank alcohol as normal (3–4 glasses of wine 2–3 times a week) until recently, when I found out I was pregnant after a positive urine pregnancy test at 6 weeks.

I have had no pv bleeding and no abdominal pain and I have not yet had an ultrasound scan to confirm my dates. This was a planned pregnancy, and we are both delighted but a little nervous about things. I have had no previous medical problems and no previous surgery other than ERPC. I have been taking folic acid for the last 6 months but no other medication. My father has diabetes for which he takes injections, but there are no other family illnesses.

Assessment	Good	Adequate	Poor/Not Done
1 Appropriate introduction (full name and role)	☐	☐	☐
2 Establishes reason for visit	☐	☐	☐
3 Establishes:			
LNMP		☐	☐
Regular 28 day cycle		☐	☐
Recent COCP use (up to 6 months before)		☐	☐
Whether had dating scan (no) Symptoms of early pregnancy	☐	☐	☐
(nausea and vomiting, breast tenderness, frequency) Confirmation (+ve test at 6 weeks)	☐	☐	☐
Any problems (pv bleeding, pain)	☐	☐	☐
Any current medications	☐	☐	☐
4 Establishes history of previous pregnancies (number = 1)		☐	☐
Duration of pregnancy (8/40)		☐	☐
Outcome (miscarriage needing ERPC)	☐	☐	☐
5 Establishes past medical history:			
Major medical illnesses and treatment (nil)	☐	☐	☐
Surgical operations (nil)	☐	☐	☐
Gynaecological problems (nil)	☐	☐	☐
Last cervical smear (1 year, normal)	☐	☐	☐
Drug history (folic acid only)	☐	☐	☐
Family history (father IDDM)	☐	☐	☐

6 Establishes whether the patient works and if so, what kind of work   ☐   ☐   ☐

7 Establishes if the patient is married or in long-term relationship:

   Smoking history (no)   ☐   ☐

   Alcohol (moderate usage now stopped)   ☐   ☐   ☐

8 Elicits patient's concerns and responds sensitively   ☐   ☐   ☐

9 Appropriate questioning technique.   ☐   ☐   ☐

10 Avoids or explains jargon   ☐   ☐   ☐

11 Summarises history back to patient, including concerns   ☐   ☐   ☐

12 Systematic, organised approach   ☐   ☐   ☐

SP to mark

13 The doctor was empathic   ☐   ☐   ☐

Comment

The history must include:

- Accurate menstrual history (LNMP and cycle length), early US (or not) to confirm or change dates, pregnancy confirmation (test), symptoms of early pregnancy and any common problems, eg bleeding or pain.
- All previous pregnancies (full term, TOPs, miscarriages, ectopics), duration, outcome, complications, mode of delivery, birthweight, type of feeding.
- Past gynaecological (including cervical smear) and medical history and family history of heart disease, hypertension and diabetes.
- Home circumstances and occupational/lifestyle (smoking and alcohol) history.
- Fertility treatment, multiple pregnancies and/or birth defects may be relevant.

The whole point of the history is to identify any risk factors for the current pregnancy that need to be either monitored or acted upon to try and optimise the outcome for mother and baby.

Answers

STATION 2.2

Patient History

I have not seen my periods for 6 weeks and am worried that I am pregnant, as I did not plan to be and it would be a disaster as my job is so busy. My periods have been 28 days and regular since stopping the COCP 5 months ago. I had been on the contraceptive pill for the past 5 years or so but came off it 5 months ago because I had broken up with my long-term boyfriend and no longer needed contraception. I am single and have no current regular partner. I had sex with a condom last month but we didn't use it at all times. I didn't have time to get the emergency pill as I went abroad with my job straight after. I work full-time as a producer for a local TV and cable company.

My breasts feel full and sore at present, and I feel sick in the mornings. I am getting up at night to pass water and am going more frequently during the day. I have had no pv bleeding, discharge or pain. I have not done a test yet as I've been too scared to get the answer.

I have had a termination of pregnancy at about 8 weeks when I was 17 years old but no other pregnancies. My last smear was 2 years ago (normal) and I have never had any sexually transmitted infections. I have always been healthy and fit and have no other medical or family history of note. I do not smoke but drink 'quite heavily' mainly at the weekend.

Assessment	Good	Adequate	Poor/not done
1 Appropriate introduction (full name and role)	☐	☐	☐
2 Elucidates reason for visit	☐	☐	☐
3 Establishes: Symptoms of early pregnancy			
(nausea and vomiting, breast tenderness, frequency)	☐	☐	☐
Confirmation test (no)		☐	☐
Any problems (PV bleeding, discharge, pain – no)	☐	☐	☐

4 Establishes:
LNMP ☐ ☐

Regular 28 day cycle ☐ ☐

Recent COCP use (up to 5 months before) ☐ ☐ ☐

Recent sexual contact and contraceptive
practice (condom but not always) ☐ ☐ ☐

Use of emergency contraception (no) ☐ ☐ ☐

5 Previous termination history ☐ ☐ ☐

6 Establishes attitude to pregnancy/need
for counselling ('disaster'/yes) ☐ ☐ ☐

7 Establishes gynaecological history:
(smear, sexually transmitted infection) ☐ ☐ ☐

8 Establishes current and past general
health any current medications (nil)

Alcohol consumption/smoking ☐ ☐ ☐

Family and social history ☐ ☐ ☐

9 Elicits patient's concerns and responds
sensitively ☐ ☐ ☐

10 Appropriate questioning technique. ☐ ☐ ☐

11 Avoids or explains jargon ☐ ☐ ☐

12 Summarises history back to patient,
including concerns ☐ ☐ ☐

13 Systematic, organised approach ☐ ☐ ☐

SP to mark

14 The doctor was empathic ☐ ☐ ☐

Answers

Comment

The patient is anxious and worried, and pregnancy is highly likely given her symptoms and the fact that she has had some unprotected intercourse. It does, however, need confirmation by urinary HCG test (+/- US if any doubt). She must, therefore, be questioned sympathetically, and she should develop confidence that she would be supported and cared for in her present situation and offered all possible options.

STATION 2.3

Patient History

This news is what I was afraid of and the timing is 'all wrong' for lots of reasons, including not having a steady partner and a very busy work schedule. My work involves a good deal of foreign travel, and I have a full-work schedule for the next year or so. Taking time off for this would mean professional sacrifices and I am confused and unable to decide right now, but need your advice and help in arriving at a decision.

I may think of going through with the pregnancy, but if I decide on a termination how much time do I have? Would it affect my health in any way? As I have had a previous termination does this mean I will have a problem having children later in life when I want to?

I have not told my partner, a work colleague, who is responsible for my pregnancy, and I do not want him to be involved in any decisions I make as it was only a casual relationship. However, my best friend Julia is aware and is a great help to talk to. There is nobody else, eg family I could possibly discuss this with.

If offered I would also welcome the chance to talk to a counsellor about my options.

I had not considered the possibility of sexually transmitted infection but think it would be sensible to have a check-up, just in case.

Assessment	Good	Adequate	Poor/Not done
1 Tells patient that she is pregnant	☐	☐	☐
2 Establishes patient's initial reactions	☐	☐	☐
3 Establishes patient's concerns.	☐	☐	☐
4 Will male partner be informed/involved (no)	☐	☐	☐
Any other support available (friend/family)	☐	☐	☐
5 Explains antenatal support during pregnancy and social service support following birth if required	☐	☐	☐
6 Explains procedures for surgical and medical termination of pregnancy (timing <13/40 surgical, <9/40 medical)	☐	☐	☐

7 Explains that termination in first
  trimester is done as a day procedure and
  carries low risks to health and fertility ☐   ☐   ☐

8 Second termination not usually a problem
  for future fertility but if decides on TOP
  needs to have future contraceptive advice
  Offers STI screening   ☐   ☐   ☐

9 Offers further counselling to discuss
  options   ☐   ☐   ☐

10 Offers to counsel patient and partner
   if this is wanted   ☐   ☐   ☐

11 Empathic and non-judgemental   ☐   ☐   ☐

Comment

The doctor has to guide the patient through a highly emotive and sensitive decision-making process with underlying socio-religious implications. It is important to check whether she has support from either a partner, friend or family member(s) to help her make a decision now she knows she is pregnant.

Counselling of the patient (+/- her partner) should be directed towards the support available to take her safely through her pregnancy, or on the safety/risks of pregnancy termination. The doctor should refrain from expressing his/her personal, moral or ethical views.

Other areas that must be addressed are whether she wishes to have STI screening as she is at risk future contraception if she decides on a TOP; and the offer of further skilled early pregnancy counselling.

STATION 2.4a

Patient History

I have always been fit and well, although overweight. I am 1.54m and 80 kilograms. I am 28 weeks pregnant with my first child. I have come for the results of a glucose tolerance test I had 5 days ago. This was a routine test 'that everyone gets' and I am concerned that it shows I have diabetes. Though concerned, I am not entirely surprised as my father, aged 55, has diabetes, that is controlled with diet and tablets.

I have stopped smoking and drinking alcohol since finding out that I am pregnant but I have 'a very sweet tooth' and would appreciate some advice about my diet (if offered). Nobody has explained the results or the implications and I have no concept of what this will mean to me or the baby. Apart from a bit of morning sickness very early on, I have been well in the last few weeks.

Assessment	Good	Adequate	Poor/Not done
1 Appropriate introduction (full name and role)	☐	☐	☐
2 Establishes patient identity and explains purpose of interview	☐	☐	☐
3 Establishes patient's understanding of the investigation results and diagnosis in a clear non-jargonistic manner	☐	☐	☐
4 Explains the investigation results and diagnosis	☐	☐	☐
5 Explains the implications of the diagnosis on the pregnancy	☐	☐	☐
Complications to the mother (hyperglycaemia, increased operative delivery, pre-eclampsia, future risk of diabetes)	☐	☐	☐
Complications to the fetus (macrosomia, polyhydramnios, RDS, neonatal hypoglycaemia)	☐	☐	☐
6 Explains the treatment alternatives – diet or insulin; no tablets may be used	☐	☐	☐
7 Need for combined clinic with consultant obstetrician, diabetologist and dietician	☐	☐	☐

8 Explains about regular blood glucose monitoring ☐ ☐ ☐

9 Explains need for regular ultrasound for fetal growth and liquor volume ☐ ☐ ☐

10 Invites patient's questions and answers appropriately ☐ ☐ ☐

   Checks patient's understanding of information ☐ ☐ ☐

11 Systematic, organised approach ☐ ☐ ☐

12 Gives clear, jargon-free explanation ☐ ☐ ☐

SP to mark

13 The doctor was sensitive to my concerns ☐ ☐ ☐

Diagnosis

Gestational Diabetes.

Comment

Management of diabetes during pregnancy:

Women with pre-existing diabetes should optimise their glycaemic control before pregnancy and should be cared for by an obstetrician and diabetologist.

Gestational diabetes is diabetes recognised for the first time after 20/40 gestation. It usually occurs because of diabetogenic effects of placental hormone production (oestrogen, cortisol, human placental lactogen) in susceptible women (eg obese, Asian, previous GDM).

GDM is thought to be a marker of susceptibility to type 2 DM in later life, with the 'stress' of pregnancy causing alterations in glycaemic control (a small percentage of women diagnosed as having new onset diabetes during pregnancy will already have insulin-dependent diabetes).

Patients may be managed with strict diabetic diet, but if this fails the only option is to use insulin. Patients are usually started on small doses of mixtard insulin, on a bd regimen, eg 8 units, mane, 4 units nocte. If this scheme fails to maintain normoglycaemia, a qds regimen may be adopted, using pre-meal actrapid and an evening dose of an intermediate-acting insulin. Doses are titrated upwards according to the patient's glycaemic control, which they must be taught to monitor using BM stix with home blood glucose monitoring (HBGM) up to four times a day.

Complications of hyperglycaemia during pregnancy

Maternal: Infections, eg vaginal candidiasis, UTIs

Hyperglycaemia

Pre-eclampsia and eclampsia

Increased operative delivery

Fetal: Intrauterine death and neonatal mortality are both greatly increased

Macrosomia (large baby)

Polyhydramnios

RDS

Neonatal hypoglycaemia and jaundice

STATION 2.5a

Patient History

I am 42 years old and have always been fit and well and am 34 weeks pregnant with my first child. I have had no other pregnancies. I am fit and well and have never had problems with my blood pressure before.

I was told by the GP that my blood pressure was slightly high but I have been taking it easy and feel fine. I realise I may have to be admitted to hospital but am not very keen because I want everything to be natural if possible. I do not really understand the implications of raised blood pressure in pregnancy but have become anxious about it. My partner is very supportive but works 6 days a week and at present cannot afford to take time off.

Assessment	Good	Adequate	Poor/Not done
1 Appropriate introduction (full name and role)	☐	☐	☐
2 Establishes patient's understanding of her blood pressure problem and its implications	☐	☐	☐
3 Establishes no previous history of hypertension	☐	☐	☐
4 Enquires about PET symptoms (headache, visual disturbance, epigastric pain)	☐	☐	☐
5 Explains the risk to mother (eclampsia, renal failure, liver damage, bleeding)	☐	☐	☐
Explains the risk to fetus (poor growth, reduced liquor, abruption)	☐	☐	☐
Reassures mother that serious complicationss are uncommon if well monitored	☐	☐	☐
6 Explains that patient requires admission – monitoring + possible treatment of blood pressure, blood and urine tests, ultrasound for growth and liquor	☐	☐	☐
7 Explains delivery is curative and may need early delivery (IOL usually or LSCS)	☐	☐	☐

8 Establishes and discusses reasons why patient is reluctant to be admitted	☐	☐	☐
9 Gives clear, jargon-free explanation	☐	☐	☐
10 Checks patient's understanding of information	☐	☐	☐
11 Invites patient's questions and answers appropriately	☐	☐	☐
12 Systematic, organised approach	☐	☐	☐

SP to mark

13 The student was empathic	☐	☐	☐

Diagnosis

Likely pre-eclampsia – requires admission.

Comment

Pre-eclampsia is one of the leading causes of maternal mortality in the UK. Possible crises include: eclampsia, elevated liver enzymes and low platelets, HELLP syndrome, placental abruption, renal +/or hepatic failure and cerebral haemorrhage. The spectrum of the condition includes utero-placental insufficiency and intrauterine growth restriction with reduced liquor volume.

The patient requires admission for close monitoring of the blood pressure, FBC, U+E and urate, LFTs, clotting, 24-hour urinary protein and US and CTG for fetal well-being. Indications for delivery (the only cure) include: fetal compromise, inability to control maternal blood pressure, increasingly abnormal blood parameters and the development of maternal symptoms suggesting impending crisis, eg right upper quadrant pain, confusion, 'flashing lights', severe headache.

STATION 2.6

Assessment	Good	Adequate	Poor/Not done
1 Appropriate introduction (full name and role)	☐	☐	☐
2 Explains what interview is to be about	☐	☐	☐
3 Explains the ultrasound in appropriate detail; risk to mother and fetus is heavy but unpredictable vaginal bleeding	☐	☐	☐
4 Explains the need for delivery by caesarean section at 38–39 weeks in absence of bleeding	☐	☐	☐
5 Explains increased risk of heavy haemorrhage at CS and possible need for blood transfusion	☐	☐	☐
6 Explains need for admission in case has pv bleeding	☐	☐	☐
OR			
May stay at home as asymptomatic and have NO bleeding as long as has suitable Support	☐	☐	☐
7 Gives clear, jargon-free explanation	☐	☐	☐
8 Invites patient's questions and answers appropriately	☐	☐	☐
9 Systematic, organised approach	☐	☐	☐

Answers

Comment

Placenta praevia describes the condition where the placenta lies in the lower uterine segment. It is associated with multiple pregnancy, an abnormally large placenta, eg diabetes mellitus, uterine structural abnormalities, and previous uterine surgery, eg caesarean section. The major risk to mother and fetus is unpredictable heavy pv bleeding, requiring urgent delivery. Opinions differ as to whether asymptomatic women should be admitted after 34 weeks until delivery – either option is acceptable as long as they have no bleeding and have reliable, fast access to hospital in the event of pv bleeding.

Classification: Minor–The lower margins of the placenta not within 2 cm from
                    the cervical os.
                    Vaginal delivery may be possible.
              Major–The lower margins cover the os or are less than 2 cm
                    from the cervical os.
                    Caesarean section indicated.

STATION 2.7

Patient History

My baby is due in 2 months time and I hear that it is always difficult and painful with the first baby. I cannot stand much pain and the thought of a difficult labour is very frightening. I need to know how you are going to deal with the pain, because I want to feel as little pain as possible during labour. My sister had a long and difficult labour last year and had to have stitches. As my mum also had problems, I am scared that this may run in the family. What are my options during labour?

Assessment	Good	Adequate	Poor/Not done
1 Appropriate introduction (full name and role)	☐	☐	☐
2 Checks what patient wishes to discuss	☐	☐	☐
3 Elicits patient's concerns about labour	☐	☐	☐
4 Establishes whether patient has discussed her concerns with anyone else	☐	☐	☐
5 Establishes patient's understanding of analgesic options for childbirth	☐	☐	☐
6 Establishes whether the patient or her partner attends antenatal classes or group therapy sessions, where labour is explained, to reduce fear and anxiety	☐	☐	☐
7 Reassures that every labour experience is unique and does not run in the family	☐	☐	☐
8 Reassures the patient that complete analgesia is often achieved by epidural block, always available in the labour room	☐	☐	☐
9 Reassures the patient that epidurals are both common and safe with few side-effects	☐	☐	☐
10 Discusses other possible analgesic options (TENS, Entonox, opioids, relaxation techniques)	☐	☐	☐

11 Does all in an empathetic and professional manner	☐	☐	☐
12 Invites patient's questions and answers appropriately	☐	☐	☐
13 Systematic, organised approach	☐	☐	☐

Comment

Other forms of pain relief available are:

Transdermal electrical nerve stimulation (TENS): surface electrodes placed on a patient's back and used in early labour: the strength and frequency of impulses can be adjusted for comfort.

Opiate: pethidine IM or morphine or diamorphine IV during prolonged labour.

Inhalation analgesia: Entonox by face mask is controlled by the patient.

All the evidence suggests that the most effective form of analgesia is in fact a highly supportive and enthusiastic midwife and hence the importance of antenatal contact with midwives for adequate preparation for labour.

STATION 2.8

Assessment	Good	Adequate	Poor/not done
1 Appropriate introduction (name and role)	☐	☐	☐
2 Explains purpose and method of antenatal examination to patient	☐	☐	☐
3 Comments on external signs of pregnancy – *abdominal distension, linea nigra, striae gravidarum, fetal movements, any scars, everted umbilicus*	☐	☐	☐
Palpates abdomen for:			
4 Uterine size (correctly measures symphysiofundal height to within 3 cm)	☐	☐	☐
5 Fetal Lie	☐	☐	☐
6 Presentation	☐	☐	☐
7 Check engagement in fifths	☐	☐	☐
8 Auscultates fetal heart rate	☐	☐	☐
9 Explains findings to examiner	☐	☐	☐
10 Does all of the above in a fluent and professional manner	☐	☐	☐
Examiner questions:			
What other checks would you perform at an antenatal examination?			
11 Pallor, oedema	☐	☐	☐
12 BP and urine	☐	☐	☐

Answers

Comment

The main purpose of antenatal examinations in the vast majority of cases is to monitor normal physiology and provide reassurance and support.

Clinical abnormalities that may be commonly deteceted are anaemia, hypertension (diastolic BP of > 90 mm Hg), proteinuria or glycosuria, abnormalities in fetal growth (IUGR or macrosomia), liquor volume (oligo/polyhydramnios) or fetal lie (breech, oblique, transverse).

STATION 2.9

Assessment	Good	Adequate	Poor/Not done
1 fig 2.9a: Normal baseline rate (140 bpm), Normal baseline variability (5–25beats), Three accelerations present, No decelerations, minimal uterine activity Good = all 5 parameter Adequate = 3/4 correct Poor = 1/2 correct	☐	☐	☐
2 Normal CTG	☐	☐	☐
3 fig 2.9b: Normal baseline rate (140–150 bpm), Normal baseline variability (5–25beats), No accelerations present, type 1 or early decelerations, uterine activity 4 in 10 min.	☐	☐	☐
4 Early decelerations owing to compression of the fetal head or cord during contractions.	☐	☐	☐
5 fig 2.9c Normal baseline rate (130 bpm), Reduced baseline variability (< 5 beats), No accelerations present, No decelerations, uterine activity 3 in 10 min.	☐	☐	☐
6. Reduced variability of foetal heart rate (flat CTG) during labour due to sleep pattern, maternal opiates or possible fetal distress	☐	☐	☐

Comment

Cardiotocography in labour is used to monitor women at high risk. It is not advocated for low-risk women as it has not been shown to reduce perinatal morbidity and mortality and in fact increases the rate of operative delivery. The normal fetal heart rate in the waking state shows normal baseline rate (110–150bpm), normal baseline variability (5–25 beats) owing to normal physiological stimuli, accelerations (increase > 15 bpm for > 15 secs) and no decelerations (decrease > 15bpm for > 15 secs) as in fig 2.9a. Reduced variability results in a flat trace, showing a heart not responding to such stimuli (fig 2.9c). These variations may be caused by hypoxaemia because of reduction in placental blood flow. Sleep patterns and opiates also produce similar patterns which revert to normal in time.

Answers

STATION 2.10

	Apgar scores		
	0	**1**	**2**
Colour	Blue or pale	Blue extremities	Completely pink
Heart rate	Absent	<100/min	>100/min
Respiratory effort	Absent	Irregular	Good/crying
Muscle tone	Limp	Some flexion	Active movement
Reflex response	Absent	Minimal	Normal

Comment

The Apgar score denotes neonatal condition at birth and allows comparison of condition over time as well as giving a guide to the need for rescusitation and possible prognosis. The need for immediate resuscitatory measures and/or transfer to an intensive care unit for monitoring is indicated by an Apgar score of 7 or less. Immediately life-threatening abnormalities may also be detected during the examination.

STATION 2.11

Assessment	Good	Adequate	Poor/not done
1 General inspection: face and eyes	☐	☐	☐
2 Examination of mouth, ears and neck	☐	☐	☐
3 Examination of head and back	☐	☐	☐
4 Examination of chest and peripheral pulses	☐	☐	☐
5 Examination of abdomen, external genitalia, anus, hips and legs	☐	☐	☐
6 Does all in an efficient and professional manner	☐	☐	☐

Comment

Looks for obvious general abnormalities and assesses alertness, posture, movement and reflexes, eye abnormalities, infection and movement, and facial features suggestive of chromosomal abnormalities.

Examines mouth to exclude palatal and glossal abnormalities. External ear and mental defects, thyroid enlargement, sternomastoid tumour.

Palpates fontenelles, checks for scalp haematoma (chignon), measures head circumference, examines back for signs of neural cord defects.

Auscultates for heart murmurs and breath sounds, examines for chest wall abnormalities, eg pectus excavatum, clavicular dislocation. Absent peripheral pulses suggest aortic coarctation.

Abdomen: normal to feel liver edge, kidneys/spleen; check cord stump, exclude exomphalos and imperforate anus.

External genitalia: in male: hypospadias, testicular descent. In female: labial fusion.

Lower limbs: congenital hip dislocation, talipes.

STATION 2.12

Assessment	Good	Adequate	Poor/not done
1 Tilt manikin head down			
Aspirate airway; 100% O_2 by face mask	☐	☐	☐
2 Monitor heart rate, if rate <100/min, intubate and ventilate			
Set up venous access via umbilical vein	☐	☐	☐
3 In absence of heart beat after above, external cardiac massage Counteract acidosis by sodium bicarbonate (5 mmol/Kg wt) via umbilical vein catheter	☐	☐	☐
4 Keep neonate warm with heating pad and space blanket	☐	☐	☐
5 Does all in an efficient and professional manner	☐	☐	☐

Comment

The long-held assumption that acidosis complicates cardiac arrest and may perpetuate arrhythmias has recently been challenged. Acidosis as measured by arterial and/or central venous blood gases probably bears little relationship to myocardial intra-cellular values; the passage of carbon dioxide across the cell membrane can lower intracellular pH, while the alkaline residue of the metabolised bicarbonate increases the extracellular pH. The development of an iatrogenic alkalosis may be even less favourable than the metabolic acidosis to the myocardium; and there is no good empirical evidence in favour of sodium bicarbonate during the early stages of cardiac arrest.

Answers

STATION 2.13

Patient History

I was previously a fit and well 19-year-old engineering student. I started having periods aged 11–12 years old and these have been regular until they stopped 8 months ago. Previously, my normal cycle was 3–5/28 and regular. I am in a long-term relationship with my boyfriend and we use condoms. I have never been on the OCP.

I have never been pregnant, nor had a smear test and have not had any other gynaecological problems. I have been relatively well, but have lost 5 kilogrammes over the last year as I do a lot of sport (1–2 hours in the gym every day). I do not feel particularly stressed and am enjoying university. I have not noticed any excess hair, acne or milk leakage from my breasts.

I do not smoke and I drink 20–30 units of alcohol per week. I am not on any regular medication and have had no serious personal or family illnesses.

Assessment	Good	Adequate	Poor/not done
1 Appropriate introduction (full name and role)	☐	☐	☐
2 Explains purpose of interview and gains consent	☐	☐	☐
3 Establishes age of menarche	☐	☐	☐
4 Establishes normal menstrual cycle and last normal cycle	☐	☐	☐
5 Asks about sexual activity – establishes last sexual intercourse/excludes symptoms of pregnancy	☐	☐	☐
6 Establishes present method of contraception	☐	☐	☐
7 Establishes previous pregnancy history	☐	☐	☐
8 Establishes/excludes other gynaecological symptoms – dyspaeunia, pelvic pain	☐	☐	☐

9 Establishes/excludes symptoms of
   differential causes:

   Gross weight loss –

   (Anorexia/excess exercise) ☐ ☐ ☐

   Pituitary disease – headaches,

   visual disturbance, galactorrhoea

   PLOS (polycystic ovary syndrome) ☐ ☐ ☐

   Weight gain, acne and hirsutism

   general systemic disorders ☐ ☐ ☐

   Thyroid disease, anaemia, diabetes ☐ ☐ ☐

10 Enquires after social history and stressors ☐ ☐ ☐

11 Establishes smoking and alcohol history ☐ ☐ ☐

12 Establishes not on any medications ☐ ☐ ☐

13 Elicits patient's concerns and responds
   sensitively ☐ ☐ ☐

14 Appropriate questioning technique ☐ ☐ ☐

15 Avoids or explains jargon ☐ ☐ ☐

16 Summarises history back to patient,
   including concerns ☐ ☐ ☐

17 Systematic, organised approach ☐ ☐ ☐

18 Gives appropriate differential diagnosis.
   Excessive exercise and weight loss
   (hypothalamic amenorrhoea) ☐ ☐ ☐

Answers

Diagnosis

Secondary amenorrhoea can be due to many causes (eg PCOS, premature ovarian
failure, prolactinoma, cervical stenosis, thyroid disease), but is very common in
young women who exercise excessively, have eating disorders or may have concerns
such as a university course and relationship problems. This is thought to be
modulated via hypothalamic reduction in GnRH production.

STATION 2.14

Patient History (from wife)

I am 34 and my husband is 36 years old. We have been married for 3 years and have been trying to conceive since then. My last normal menstrual period was 1 week ago. We have sexual intercourse two or three times a week. We both work: he as a solicitor, and I am an estate agent. We own the house we live in and have no financial worries. My husband has a 5-year-old child from a previous marriage, whom he supports. And to my knowledge has had no testicular operations or trauma. I have never been pregnant and we are both healthy and fit. I had an operation for an ovarian cyst 5 years ago, when my right ovary was removed. My periods were regular when I was on the Pill, but since I came off it over 2 years ago when we started trying for a baby, they come every 6–8 weeks or so and are occasionally heavy. My last cervical smear was 1 year ago and was normal and I have never had any sexually transmitted diseases.

I have no other gynaecological history of note. We are both non-smokers, take no medication and drink three to four glasses of wine each week.

Assessment	Good	Adequate	Poor/not done
1 Appropriate introduction (full name and role)	☐	☐	☐
2 Establishes purpose of interview	☐	☐	☐
3 Establishes duration of trying to conceive	☐	☐	☐
4 Establishes history of previous pregnancies	☐	☐	☐
5 Establishes if there are any children from previous relationships	☐	☐	☐
6 Establishes LNMP and menstrual history	☐	☐	☐
7 Establishes/eliminates known gynaecological history (STIs, fibroids endometriosis)	☐	☐	☐
8 Establishes previous right oopherectomy due to ovarian cyst	☐	☐	☐
9 Establishes past/present health of husband	☐	☐	☐

10 Establishes frequency of sexual intercourse	☐	☐	☐
11 Asks about occupations of couple and home circumstances	☐	☐	☐
12 Establishes smoking and alcohol for both partners	☐	☐	☐
13 Appropriate questioning technique without jargon and with organised and empathetic approach	☐	☐	☐

Answers

Comment

Fertility problems should be considered a couple's problem, rather than individual within a relationship. Subfertility should only be diagnosed after the couple have been having a full sexual relationship for 1 year. After the initial interview with the couple together, it may be appropriate to interview them separately, but all management decisions should be made in open discussion and with the agreement of both partners.

The loss of an ovary only slightly reduces the chances of normal conception and menstrual irregularities usually reflect anovulation (intermittent or complete) because of common endocrinopathies such as PCOS. Endocrine therapy may stimulate normal ovulation and conception, provided there are no tubal or seminal abnormalities. In-vitro fertilization (IVF) may be considered when there is prolonged subfertility and no cause is found.

STATION 2.15

Patient History

I am married and work as an actress in theatre and TV productions. I want to have my tubes tied, as we have two children, aged 8 and 10, both by normal delivery. They are fit and well. We are absolutely certain our family is complete. My job involves a good deal of time away from home, and involves working on productions in Europe.

I have had one other pregnancy resulting in an early termination 3 years ago. I am currently on the combined pill but have been taking it for years and wish to stop and get something permanent so I do not have to worry about getting pregnant any more. My GP has also discussed this with me and supports our decision.

My partner is certain he does not want to be sterilised and I am happy to be the one. I am otherwise fit and well and have had no other illnesses or medical problems before and take no medication other than my pill. I do not smoke and only drink alcohol occasionally.

Assessment	Good	Adequate	Poor/not done
1 Appropriate introduction (full name and role)	☐	☐	☐
2 Establishes purpose of interview	☐	☐	☐
3 Establishes social history	☐	☐	☐
4 Establishes reasons for wanting sterilisation	☐	☐	☐
5 Establishes current contraceptive use and reason for change	☐	☐	☐
6 Establishes past obstetric history	☐	☐	☐
7 Establishes past gynaecological and medical history	☐	☐	☐
8 Enquires into certainty of her and husband's wishes and the possibility of wanting children in the future	☐	☐	☐

9 Informs about irreversibility and future regret   ☐   ☐   ☐

   Failure rate (2/100)   ☐   ☐

   Risks of laparoscopy   ☐   ☐

   Male sterilisation safer and smaller failure rate   ☐   ☐   ☐

10 Summarises history back to patient, including concerns about health   ☐   ☐   ☐

11 Systematic, organised approach   ☐   ☐   ☐

Comment

Counselling for sterilisation for all women should explore the possibilities of a change of mind in the future, as a result of changes in social or economic circumstances or injury or illness of current children. The stability of personal relationships and socio-economic factors affecting the patient should also be explored as these groups have been shown to have high levels of regret in later life. It is mandatory to inform them of the irreversibility, failure rate of tubal ligation (1/200) and discuss the suitability of the male partner being sterilised instead, as it is technically easier, safer and has a lower failure rate (after two negative semen analyses). Major complications of laparoscopic sterilisation are rare (bowel/bladder perforation, haemorrhage, infection). These must be discussed for the patient to make a fully informed decision.

STATION 2.16

Patient History

I am 35 years old and having severe lower abdominal cramps just before my periods, and they subside only when my period ends. The pain is central, severe and radiates to my back. I have to spend the worst day or two in bed. I am single and work as a flight attendant and am having to alter my work schedule virtually every month as a result. I take paracetamol but it does not help. My periods are regular, every 28 days, and not heavy. I have been off the contraceptive pill for over a year (now using condoms) but my symptoms have simply got worse. I also find intercourse painful deep inside and often have to stop because of the pain.

I began my periods when I was 14 years old, but they became very painful about 9 months ago. I have never been pregnant and never had a pelvic infection. My last smear test was 3 months ago and was normal. I am a very healthy and active person and am not on any medication, except simple painkillers I take during menstruation. These are no longer effective.

I have had no problems with my bowels or passing urine and have had no previous operations or illnesses. I do not drink or smoke. I am really worried that something might be really wrong. I am also concerned about the effects on my job.

Assessment	Good	Adequate	Poor/not done
1 Appropriate introduction (full name and role)	☐	☐	☐
2 Establishes reason for patient's visit	☐	☐	☐
3 Establishes the characteristics of the pain: *Severity, site & radiation*	☐	☐	☐
Duration in relation to cycle	☐	☐	☐
Effect on daily activities	☐	☐	☐
Analgesia used	☐	☐	☐
Deep dyspareunia	☐	☐	☐
4 Establishes menstrual history	☐	☐	☐

5 Establishes gynaecological history:

   History STI/PID   ☐   ☐   ☐

   Current contraception   ☐   ☐   ☐

   COCP use   ☐   ☐   ☐

   Cervical smear   ☐   ☐   ☐

6 Establishes any past pregnancies   ☐   ☐   ☐

7 Establishes absence of bowel/urinary
   symptoms   ☐   ☐   ☐

8 Offers diagnosis – endometriosis, PID,
   adenomyosis   ☐   ☐   ☐

9 Elicits patient's concerns and responds
   sensitively   ☐   ☐   ☐

10 Avoids or explains jargon   ☐   ☐   ☐

11 Summarises history back to patient,
   including concerns   ☐   ☐   ☐

12 Systematic, organised approach   ☐   ☐   ☐

Comment

The patient probably has secondary dysmenorrhoea: this is usually associated with demonstrable pelvic pathology, ie endometriosis, pelvic inflammatory disease, ovarian cysts, adenomyosis and cervical stenosis. The dysmenorrhoea may be relieved symptomatically with NSAID analgesia, eg mefanemic acid or empirical hormonal treatment (eg COCP or progestagens), or by treatment of the underlying cause.

STATION 2.17

Patient History

I am 45 years old and have been having prolonged periods lasting for 8 days, with the passage of clots for the past 9 months. I have to change tampons over 10 times a day and sometimes flood through double protection. I have had no bleeding between periods or after intercourse. My periods are not particularly painful. I have not noticed any hot flushes or night sweats. My general health has always been good and I was on the combined pill until 1 year ago. I am currently using a 'copper coil' I had fitted at that time. I had a normal pregnancy 20 years ago and my son is fit and well. I had a cervical smear test a year ago which was normal. I take no regular medications and have had no major illnesses or operations. I currently live with my long-term partner and work in a publishing company.

Assessment	Good	Adequate	Poor/not done
1 Appropriate introduction (full name and role)	☐	☐	☐
2 Establishes reason for patient's visit	☐	☐	☐
3 Establishes menstrual history:			
Frequency		☐	☐
Duration		☐	☐
Blood loss	☐	☐	☐
Associated pain or cramps		☐	☐
Regularity		☐	☐
No IMB/PCB.	☐	☐	☐
4 Establishes gynaecological history			
IUCD use	☐	☐	☐
Last cervical smear	☐	☐	☐
Previous COCP use	☐	☐	☐
5 Establishes obstetric history	☐	☐	☐
6 Establishes current medications	☐	☐	☐
7 Establishes present health and major illnesses	☐	☐	☐

8 Establishes social and/or professional
   history

9 Offers reasonable diagnosis (IUCD,
   dysfunctional uterine bleeding, fibroids,
   endometrial polyp/hyperplasia)

10 Appropriate questioning technique

11 Avoids or explains jargon

12 Summarises history back to patient,
    including concerns

13 Systematic, organised approach

Diagnosis
Menorrhagia.

Comment
The normal menopause is signalled by reduced periods, with increasing intervals
between them. Dysfunctional uterine bleeding is the commonest cause and usually
presents in the climacteric. It is a diagnosis of exclusion once endometrial pathology
(polyp, hyperplasia, carcinoma) has been ruled out. IUCD use and submucosal
fibroids are other common causes.

Answers

STATION 2.18

Patient History

I am a sales representative with a marketing firm, and my work involves travelling and meeting clients. I have been constantly staining my underwear for the past 6 months or so, with itching of the surrounding skin; this is embarrassing when I am in company. The discharge is whitish, and does not smell. I have to wash and change my underwear constantly to be hygienic.

My periods started when I was 14 and are regular. I have had no bleeding between periods or after intercourse. My periods are not particularly painful. I had a cervical smear test a year ago which was normal.

I had a termination of pregnancy about 8 years ago when I was at college but have had no other pregnancies. I have never had any sexually transmitted or pelvic infections to my knowledge, nor have I attended a 'sexual health' clinic. I've been on the combined pill for many years and I started a new relationship about 8–9 months ago. I take no regular medications and have had no major illnesses or operations.

I am very anxious to be sorted out.

Assessment	Good	Adequate	Poor/not done
1 Appropriate introduction (full name and role)	☐	☐	☐
2 Explains purpose of interview	☐	☐	☐
3 Characteristics of discharge:			
Colour		☐	☐
Odour		☐	☐
Quantity (Number of pads used)		☐	☐
Associated itching/irritation	☐	☐	☐
4 O & G history:			
Age at menarche		☐	☐
Cervical smear	☐	☐	☐
Menstrual problems	☐	☐	☐
STI/Pelvic infections	☐	☐	☐
Use of contraception	☐	☐	☐
Pregnancy history	☐	☐	☐
Attendance at a GU clinic	☐	☐	☐

5 Current sexual partner – how long
   together, any other partners   ☐   ☐   ☐

6 Reasonable diagnosis (candida, STI,
   eg chlamydia, local cause, eg cervical
   polyp/carcinoma, ectropion)   ☐   ☐   ☐

7 Elicits patient's concerns and responds
   sensitively   ☐   ☐   ☐

8 Appropriate questioning techinique   ☐   ☐   ☐

9 Avoids or explains jargon   ☐   ☐   ☐

10 Summarises history back to patient,
    including concerns   ☐   ☐   ☐

11 Systematic, organised approach   ☐   ☐   ☐

SP to mark

12 The student was easy to talk to   ☐   ☐   ☐

Comment

The aetiological factors for the type of discharge the patient describes are:

- Vaginal infections, eg candida/bacterial vaginosis.
- Local cervical cause, eg cervical polyp/carcinoma, ectropion – use of the contraceptive pill commonly causes ectropion.
- STIs, eg chlamydia, gonorrhoea, trichomonas.

The last requires information on sexual exposure, previous episodes and treatment and whether the patient had attended a GU clinic.

Answers

STATION 2.19

Patient History

I am a school teacher, and am returning for the results of a cervical smear test I had several weeks ago. My previous smear, 5 years ago, was normal, and I have no anxieties about the results of this test.

(When told about the results)

I am very concerned about what you've just said:

Does this mean I have cancer?

What will happen when I go to the hospital?

Assessment	Good	Adequate	Poor/Not done
1 Appropriate introduction (full name and role)	☐	☐	☐
2 Establishes reason for attendance	☐	☐	☐
3 Explains purpose of interview	☐	☐	☐
4 Explains the results of the smear test, communicating appropriately, the seriousness of the condition: This is NOT cancer but pre-malignant. If left long term there is a significant risk of cancer – needs prompt treatment	☐	☐	☐
5 Explains the need for colposcopy and biopsy to confirm diagnosis	☐	☐	☐
6 Explains the procedure for colposcopy: Outpatient procedure Similar to normal smear except for use of colposcope Biopsy usually causes minimal discomfort	☐	☐	☐
7 Mentions likely need for local treatment of the cervix (loop excision, cone biopsy, laser, cold or hot coagulation): Outpatient or day-case	☐	☐	☐

Answers

8 Explains need for follow-up after
   treatment with smears annually   ☐   ☐   ☐

9 Gives clear, jargon-free explanation ☐   ☐   ☐

10 Gives appropriate reassurance   ☐   ☐   ☐

11 Checks patients understanding of
   explanation   ☐   ☐   ☐

12 Invites patient questions and answers
   appropriately   ☐   ☐   ☐

13 Systematic, organised approach   ☐   ☐   ☐

SP to mark

14 The student was empathic   ☐   ☐   ☐

Comment

Severe dyskaryosis is a cytological diagnosis most likely to correspond to CIN III. Severe dyskaryosis requires colposcopy and biopsy to gain a histological confirmation of CIN III. Local treatment includes loop excision of the transformation zone (LLETZ), cryotherapy, laser treatment and cone biopsy. The patient requires annual review with cervical smears after treatment for at least 5 years. When giving the results of an abnormal cervical smear, sensitive counselling is essential to avoid emotional problems and possible delay in diagnosis and treatment.

STATION 2.20

Patient History

For the past 5 to 6 months I have a constant sensation of something dragging in the lower abdomen and a feeling of fullness in the vagina. I am in constant discomfort during the day and get backache when I am up and about; I have difficulty coping with the housework. I have five children (all were large), the first two were breech presentations with difficult births. I had no problems when the other three were born. I find that I have difficulty holding my water and occasionally wet myself if I cough or sneeze. I tend to be constipated and have to take laxatives from time to time. I had my gall bladder removed 5 years ago for gallstones but no other opertaions. I am otherwise fit and well.

My periods stopped when I was 50, I have had no vaginal bleeding since and I do not take HRT. I do not smoke and only drink occasional alcohol.

I am worried about what might be wrong and whether it can be treated. It is very embarrassing to wet myself.

Assessment	Good	Adequate	Poor/not done
1 Appropriate introduction (full name and role)	☐	☐	☐
2 Establishes reason for patient's attendance	☐	☐	☐
3 Establishes sensation of bearing down:			
Site		☐	☐
Duration		☐	☐
Whether felt a vaginal mass		☐	☐
Associated symptoms:	☐	☐	☐
Urinary tract (stress incontinence)	☐	☐	☐
Bowel (constipation)	☐	☐	☐
4 Establishes age of menopause and absence of bleeding	☐	☐	☐
5 Establishes not on HRT	☐	☐	☐

6 Obstetric history and risk factors:

   Number of children　　　　　　□　　　□　　　□

   Difficult deliveries　　　　　　□　　　□　　　□

   Large size babies.　　　　　　□　　　□　　　□

7 Past illnesses (medical & surgical)　□　　□　　□

8 Current medication　　　　　　□　　　□　　　□

9 Other risk factors: smoking　　□　　　□　　　□

10 Elicits patient's concerns and responds
    sensitively　　　　　　　　　□　　　□　　　□

11 Appropriate questioning technique　□　　□　　□

12 Avoids or explains jargon　　　□　　　□　　　□

13 Summarises history back to patient,
    including concerns　　　　　　□　　　□　　　□

14 Systematic organised approach　□　　　□　　　□

15 Makes a reasonable attempt at the
    diagnosis (uterovaginal prolapse, cystocele,
    rectocele)　　　　　　　　　□　　　□　　　□

Answers

Diagnosis
Uterovaginal prolapse.

Comment
A clinical diagnosis of uterovaginal prolapse is made on a good history and pelvic examination. Prolonged or difficult labour and delivery (especially forceps) and high birth-weight are the main predisposing factors. Other associated factors are obesity, being post-menopausal and anything that increases intra-abdominal pressure, eg constipation, chronic cough. Concurrently the adjacent bladder or rectal walls may bulge into the anterior or posterior vagina. Post-natal pelvic floor exercises help to strengthen pelvic musculature and may prevent the later development of prolapse.

Prolapse may be treated symptomatically with a vaginal pessary support. The surgical approach of vaginal hysterectomy and anterior or posterior colporrhaphy involves buttressing the anterior or posterior aspects of the pelvic floor musculature.

STATION 2.21

Assessment	Good	Adequate	Poor/not done
1 Appropriate introduction (full name and role) consent	☐	☐	☐
2 Indicates need for chaperone	☐	☐	☐
3 Candidates wash their hands using the alcohol handwash provided (no marks if candidate only expresses the need to wash if handwash is provided)	☐	☐	☐
4 Puts on gloves		☐	☐
5 Inspects the vulva commenting on appearance and any abnormalities	☐	☐	☐
6 Parts labia		☐	☐
7 Performs bimanual examination correctly	☐	☐	☐
8 Comments correctly on:			
Position of the uterus		☐	☐
Size of the uterus		☐	☐
Mobility of the uterus		☐	☐
Presence or absence of adnexal pathology		☐	☐
9 Disposes of gloves into clinical waste bag	☐	☐	☐
10 Does all the above in a fluent, professional manner	☐	☐	☐

Comment

A vaginal examination requires sensitivity, gentleness and skill. It is carried out in the presence of a chaperone, after counselling the patient, in a private environment. The examination gives access to all pelvic organs and enables you to assess their consistency, size and mobility, and the origin of any pelvic pathology.

STATION 2.22

Assessment	Good	Adequate	Poor/Not done
1 Appropriate introduction (full name and role)	☐	☐	☐
2 Explanation and consent	☐	☐	☐
3 Indicates need for chaperone	☐	☐	☐
4 Candidates wash their hands using the alcohol handwash provided (no marks if candidate only expresses the need to wash if handwash is provided)	☐	☐	☐
5 Checks all items required to take smear are present – speculum, microscope slide, fixative, Ayre's spatula, pencil (fig 2.22)	☐	☐	☐
6 Candidate mentions information that needs to go on slide (name of patient, date, hospital number in pencil)	☐	☐	☐
7 Puts on gloves		☐	☐
8 Positions patient	☐	☐	☐
9 Ensures speculum is warm and in working order	☐	☐	☐
10 Examines vulva and comments on appearance	☐	☐	☐
11 Parts labia and inserts speculum correctly	☐	☐	☐
12 Locks speculum with cervix well demonstrated	☐	☐	☐
13 Inserts smear spatula and rotates through 360º of the cervix	☐	☐	☐
14 Spreads smear over the microscope slide and fixes it correctly using fixative	☐	☐	☐
15 Gently closes and removes speculum	☐	☐	☐
16 Disposes of speculum into sterile services bag	☐	☐	☐

17 Disposes of gloves into clinical waste bag   ☐   ☐   ☐

18 Does all the above in a fluent, professional
    manner   ☐   ☐   ☐

Comment

Cervical screening is one of two current UK population screening programmes (the other being mammography). Cervical smears must be obtained and fixed in the prescribed manner to obviate variations in technique for the cytologist to accurately interpret cellular changes of dyskaryosis (mild, moderate, severe = CIN I,II,III) and occasionally frank malignancy.

STATION 2.23

1 fig 2.23a: *Trichomonas vaginalis*
  fig 2.23b: *Candida albicans*
2 Fresh smear from a high vaginal swab, diluted with normal saline and spread on a slide with a coverslip, and examined microscopically for TV. Direct microscopy of discharge may show candida.
3 Fig 2.23a: metronidazole (400 mg tds orally for 7 days). Also treat the partner.
  Fig 2.23b: Topical anti-fungal agents: clotrimazole, miconazole or nystatin in the form of pessaries and cream.
4 TV is sexually transmitted. Thrush (monilia) is associated with pregnancy, diabetes, oral contraceptive use or oestrogen therapy and occasionally as a superinfection following prolonged antibiotic therapy.

STATION 2.24

1 Hysterosalpingogram.
2 Infertility due to tubal abnormalities eg endometriosis, PID or structural uterine abnomalities, eg septum, bicornuate uterus, intracavity fibroids.
3 A: Uterus; B: Fallopian tube.
4 The patient is positioned in the lithotomy position on the X-ray table and the cervix exposed by means of a bivalve speculum. A cannula is introduced into the cervix and contrast medium is injected into the uterine cavity. Serial exposures of the pelvis are then taken with an image intensifier. (Patient sedation may be required.)
5 Laparoscopy and dye or hydro-contrast–sonography (Hy-Co-Sy).

Comment
Blockage or stenosis of the Fallopian tubes is a common cause of secondary infertility, resulting from chronic pelvic infection, endometriosis or previous pelvic surgery. Identifying and treating any ongoing infection may result in resolution of the inflammation and re-establishing tubal patency. Blockage caused by fibrosis and scarring is usually bypassed with in-vitro fertilisation (IVF). Tubal reconstruction may be feasible, but has a lower success rate than IVF and is highly operator dependent.

Answers

STATION 2.25

Assessment	Good	Adequate	Poor/Not done
1 Hydatitiform mole Invasive mole (chorioadenoma detruens) Choriocarcinoma (malignant trophoblastic disease) HCG-secreting tumour, eg ovarian	☐	☐	☐
2 Discrete rounded ('cannon ball') opacities in lung parenchyma Diagnosis: Pulmonary metastases from choriocarcinoma	☐	☐	☐
3 Chemotherapy usually with methotrexate alone (usually sufficient) or in combination with etoposide, cyclophosphamide and/or actinomycin D	☐	☐	☐
Local complications from a large primary tumour, such as uterine perforation or severe bleeding may require a hysterectomy	☐	☐	☐

Comment

Trophobastic disease usually follows pregnancy; a hydatidiform mole represents a chromosomally abnormal pregnancy where chorionic villi have become hydropic with trophoblastic proliferation. Complete moles usually have a complete paternally derived DNA make-up. Incomplete moles can even have some normal pregnancy features. The excessive trophoblastic proliferation can rarely become morbidly adherent to the myometrium, resulting in invasive mole (persistent trophoblastic tissue). In choriocarcinoma the trophoblastic elements have developed malignant characteristics and have a ready affinity to wide haematogenous metastases.

Diagnosis of a molar pregnancy is suggested by a rapid increase in uterine size, vaginal bleeding and/or passage of grape-like molar tissue. Confirmation is by ultrasound scanning of the uterus and elevated urinary HCG titres.

Evacuation of a hydatidiform mole following detection is followed up with serial urinary HCG measurements and chest radiographs to exclude malignant progression. Contraception is necessary over the medium term as surveillance (ie HCG measurement) may be compromised by pregnancy.

Answers

STATION 2.26

Assessment	Good	Adequate	Poor/Not done
1 Appropriate introduction (full name and role)	☐	☐	☐
2 Explains the nature of the examination	☐	☐	☐
3 Positions manikin correctly initially upright	☐	☐	☐
4 Candidate washes their hands using the alcohol handwash provided (no marks if candidate only expresses the need to wash if handwash is provided)	☐	☐	☐
Comments correctly on:			
5 Inspection for skin changes, obvious masses/asymmetry/nipple changes	☐	☐	☐
6 Presence or absence of skin or deep tethering in three arm positions (arms by side, arms above head, hands on hips)	☐	☐	☐
Procedure:			
7 Examines R and L breast with flat part of fingers, pushing the breast tissue against the chest wall	☐	☐	☐
8 Examines all four quadrants of the breasts equally well	☐	☐	☐
9 Detects any lumps	☐	☐	☐
10 Describes the nature of lumps (size, mobility, consistency, tenderness)	☐	☐	☐
11 Examines the areolae and nipples and tries to express any discharge or blood	☐	☐	☐
12 Examines the breast tails and axillae for lymphadenopathy	☐	☐	☐
13 Examines the neck from behind for cervical lymphadenopathy	☐	☐	☐

Answers

14 Indicates need to repeat the examination
supine   ☐   ☐   ☐

15 Examination undertaken in a gentle
manner   ☐   ☐   ☐

16 Candidate's technique is confident   ☐   ☐   ☐

Comment

Breast symptoms (pain, lumps, galactorrhoea) are extremely common in gynaecological patients. Most patients require help with self-examination technique or reassurance, as many patients are concerned that they may have breast cancer. This is an intimate examination and the patient's dignity needs to be maintained at all times.

Answers

STATION 2.27

Patient History

I am 25 years old and live with my partner and 2-year old daughter in a local flat. I work as a machinist in a clothes factory. We have been together since I was 19.

Gynaecological history

My periods started when I was 11 years old and were regular by the age of 13. My period lasts 4 days, every 28 days regularly. The first day of my last normal period was = 16 weeks gestation.

I have used the Pill intermittently in the past, but no contraception in the last 8 months as I was trying to conceive.

My last smear was 1 year ago – normal (and always been normal).

Obstetric history

Previous pregnancies: I had my daughter aged 23.

I had problems with blood pressure and 'protein in the water' (urine) when I was 36 weeks pregnant. At 37 weeks I was induced because of the blood pressure but had an emergency caesarean section because the 'baby got into distress'.

The baby was well and she weighed 6 lbs and has not had any problems since then.

She was bottle-fed.

Other than one complete miscarriage at 8 weeks gestation 2 years ago (no intervention required), I have had no other pregnancies.

Present situation

I did a home pregnancy urine test, when I missed my period, which was positive. I had morning nausea and my breasts were swollen and tender up till about 12 weeks.

The GP sent me to the early pregnancy confirmation clinic for a scan at 8 weeks, which confirmed my menstrual dates.

I also had a scan at 12 weeks to look at the back of the baby's neck (to check for Down's syndrome) which was normal.

I am very pleased to be pregnant and am keen to have a normal delivery if possible this time. I am well supported by my partner.

If asked:

My blood pressure has been normal since my daughter was born.

I am not taking any medications and I do not smoke or drink alcohol.

Assessment	Good	Adequate	Poor/Not done
1 Appropriate introduction (full name and role)	☐	☐	☐
2 Explains purpose of interview	☐	☐	☐
Previous obstetric history, establishes:			
3 Number of term deliveries	☐	☐	☐
4 Number of TOPs/miscarriages	☐	☐	☐
5 Need for intervention or not after miscarriage	☐	☐	☐
Previous term pregnancy, establishes:			
6 Gestation at delivery		☐	☐
7 Patient had pre-eclampsia		☐	☐
8 Patient was induced		☐	☐
9 Patient had emergency Caesarean section		☐	☐
10 Reason for Caesarean Section		☐	☐
11 Birth weight of baby		☐	☐
12 Health of baby post-delivery		☐	☐
13 Method of feeding		☐	☐
14 Blood pressure post-pregnancy		☐	☐
15 Contraception since last pregnancy	☐	☐	☐
Present pregnancy, establishes:			
16 Date of last menstrual period		☐	☐
17 Regularity of cycle		☐	☐
18 Confirmatory test + scans	☐	☐	☐
19 Symptoms of pregnancy	☐	☐	☐
20 Problems (none) in first trimester	☐	☐	☐
21 Patient's feelings about this pregnancy	☐	☐	☐
22 Appropriate questioning style	☐	☐	☐
23 Systematic and organised	☐	☐	☐

STATION 2.28

History

I am a 21-year old student. I have just started a sexual relationship with a boyfriend and have come to the FPC today for contraceptive advice. I took the pill for 2 years when I was 18 and put on a lot of weight so I am keen to try condoms. I want to make sure that I and my boyfriend know how to use a condom properly. You may find the request a bit odd, but I never had any education about it at school. As far as I am concerned, the most important thing is that you do not get pregnant.

You can talk about sex and contraception quite easily unless you are made to feel embarrassed.

The student should check that you have understood the explanation by asking you to put the condom on the condom trainer as you have been instructed.

Assessment	Good	Adequate	Poor/Not done
1 Appropriate introduction (full name and role)	☐	☐	☐
2 Checks exactly what the patient wishes to discuss	☐	☐	☐
Putting on a condom:			
3 Checks expiry date	☐	☐	☐
4 Advises application of condom *before* intercourse	☐	☐	☐
5 Squeezes teat	☐	☐	☐
6 Unrolls condom over condom trainer completely	☐	☐	☐
7 Advises against the use of oils/lubricants	☐	☐	☐
8 Advises holding on to the base of the condom when withdrawing	☐	☐	☐
9 Explains about availability of free condoms from FPC	☐	☐	☐
10 Checks understanding of condom application (asks patient to demonstrate it)	☐	☐	☐

Advice should condom break:

11 Need for emergency contraception ☐ ☐ ☐

12 Source of emergency contraception
    (GP/FPC/GUM/chemist) ☐ ☐ ☐

13 Need to take within 72 hours ☐ ☐ ☐

14 Gives clear, jargon-free explanation ☐ ☐ ☐

15 Checks whether patient has any questions ☐ ☐ ☐

16 Does not cause embarrassment ☐ ☐ ☐

Comment

Barrier contraception is a highly effective method of contraception when used correctly and also has the advantage of protection against STIs. When counselling people on the use of barrier methods a professional and clear explanation without causing embarrassment is very important. Post-coital contraception is highly effective at preventing pregnancy in the event of condom breakage as long as it is taken appropriately.

STATION 2.29

Patient history

I am 24 years old and am attending the surgery today to start taking the combined oral contraceptive pill for the first time. I am certain I want to use this method but have little prior knowledge about it.

You have come to discuss this with the GP who has asked whether you would mind talking first to a medical student who is working at the practice. You have given your consent for this. You are a matter-of-fact person who can talk about sex and contraception quite easily unless you are made to feel embarrassed.

Assessment	Good	Adequate	Poor
1 Appropriate introduction (full name and role)	☐	☐	☐
2 Checks exactly what the patient wishes to discuss including prior knowledge of pill	☐	☐	☐
Starting a pill:			
3 Start day 1 of cycle (no alternative contraception required)	☐	☐	☐
4 Start day 5 of cycle (barrier method for seven days)	☐	☐	☐
5 Take for 21 days (at same time of day).	☐	☐	☐
6 Stop for 7 day break (will have period)	☐	☐	☐
7 Start next packet after 7 day break	☐	☐	☐
Side-effects:			
8 **Minor –** irregular bleeding, simple headache, weight gain, breast tenderness	☐	☐	☐
9 Reassure most habituate	☐	☐	☐
10 **Serious –** Hypertension	☐	☐	☐
11 Focal migraine	☐	☐	☐

12 Venous thrombosis	☐	☐	☐
13 Breast cancer	☐	☐	☐
14 Reassure absolute risk is very low	☐	☐	☐

Beneficial effects:

15 Periods – less flow and pain	☐	☐	☐
16 Reduction in ovarian and endometrial cancer			
Explains missing pill protocol	☐	☐	☐
Take missed pill immediately (<12 hours no alternative contraception required)	☐	☐	☐
>12 hours take when remembered (use condoms/abstain for 7 days)	☐	☐	☐
If in last 7 days of pill packet – continue next pack without a break	☐	☐	☐
Advice as above about antibiotics	☐	☐	☐
Advice as above about diarrhoea and vomiting	☐	☐	☐

Other info:

17 Follow-up three months to check BP	☐	☐	☐
18 Operations or travel	☐	☐	☐
19 Offers written information/leaflet	☐	☐	☐
20 Checks patient understanding	☐	☐	☐
21 Invites questions	☐	☐	☐

Comment

The combined oral contraceptive pill (COCP) is a highly effective contraceptive method when used correctly. It is vital that all people about to use the COCP are aware of the current guidelines for its safe and effective usage. Serious side-effects of the pill are, in fact, rare. Users need to have all the correct information on which to make a fully informed contraceptive choice.

STATION 2.30

History

I am a 25-year old bank clerk. I am otherwise fit and well and am currently 16 weeks into my first pregnancy. Up till now there have been no problems in this pregnancy.

Last week at antenatal clinic my serum screening (blood test) for Down's syndrome gave a high-risk result of 1:80 (the normal risk at your age is 1:1500). I was told about the result 2 days ago by the midwife at the clinic and am still somewhat shocked and worried by the result. 'Does this mean my baby has Down's syndrome?' I am aware of some of the problems associated with Down's syndrome and both I and my husband have decided that we want to know for sure and would like an amniocentesis. I understand it involves putting a needle in my abdomen, but want to know more about it before you go ahead, as I am very worried it might do some harm to the baby.

I am also keen to know what options are available if the baby does have Down's syndrome.

Assessment	Good	Adequate	Poor/Not done
1 Appropriate introduction (full name and role)	☐	☐	☐
2 Explains purpose of interview	☐	☐	☐
Establishes:			
3 Patient's understanding of why amniocentesis has been offered and amniocentesis procedure	☐	☐	☐
4 Explains why procedure offered	☐	☐	☐
5 Screening high risk for Down's syndrome so diagnostic test offered to confirm/refute diagnosis	☐	☐	☐

Explains procedure:

6   Procedure involves insertion of needle
    through abdomen into amniotic sac   ☐   ☐   ☐

7   Ultrasound guidance at all times by expert ☐   ☐   ☐

8   Mild, short–lived discomfort on insertion   ☐   ☐   ☐

9   Amniotic fluid 15–20 ml withdrawn   ☐   ☐   ☐

10 Ultrasound check of fetal heart afterwards ☐   ☐   ☐

11 Go home later that day   ☐   ☐   ☐

12 Cells from fluid analysed for chromosomes   ☐   ☐   ☐

Explains complications:

13 Miscarriage 0.5–1%   ☐   ☐   ☐

14 Amniotic fluid leak/infection   ☐   ☐   ☐

15 Reassure complications rare   ☐   ☐   ☐

Explains results and limitations:

16 Two weeks for full result (cell culture)
    (extra mark if mention fast preliminary
    result within 24–48 hours)   ☐   ☐   ☐

17 Correct result 99+% (not 100%)   ☐   ☐   ☐

Explains options if positive result:

18 Enquires re patient's feelings if positive
    result   ☐   ☐   ☐

19 Emphasises full support whatever decision   ☐   ☐   ☐

20 Options involve continuation or TOP   ☐   ☐   ☐

21 Explains in a clear non-jargonistic manner ☐   ☐   ☐

22 Invites patient's questions and answers
    appropriately   ☐   ☐   ☐

Comment

Amniocentesis is usually performed for the detection of chromosomal abnormalities. Fibroblasts from the amniotic fluid are cultured for their chromosome content. Indications for amniocentesis include: high-risk serum or nuchal translucency screening, maternal age >37 and known Robertsonian translocation carrier status.

The procedure-related miscarriage risk is 0.5–1% and there is a culture failure rate of less than 1%.

Answers

STATION 2.31

History

I am a 25-year old bank clerk. I am otherwise fit and well and am currently 34 weeks into your first pregnancy. Up till now there have been no problems in this pregnancy.

Last week at antenatal clinic I was told by the midwife that my uterus was smaller than expected and that I needed a scan to check how well the baby was growing. I am aware that the scan has shown my baby is small and the fluid around it is reduced, but I want to know why this has happened and what it means for me and the baby. 'Is my baby going to be okay?' My blood pressure and urine have been okay and I am a non-smoker.

Assessment	Good	Adequate	Poor/Not done
1 Appropriate introduction (full name and role)	☐	☐	☐
2 Explains purpose of interview	☐	☐	☐
Establishes:			
3 Patient's understanding of ultrasound findings	☐	☐	☐
4 Explains scan findings.	☐	☐	☐
5 Poor fetal growth (especially abdominal)			
Reduced liquor volume	☐	☐	☐
Reduced flow in umbilical cord	☐	☐	☐
Explains significance:			
6 Findings highly suggestive of poorly functioning placenta leading to growth and fluid reduction	☐	☐	☐
7 Underlying cause uncertain	☐	☐	☐
8 May be associated with smoking and pre-eclampsia but sometimes no cause found	☐	☐	☐

Explains management:

9 Enquires about fetal movement □ □ □

10 Need for kick-chart □ □ □

11 Further fetal monitoring required –
regular CTGs

(daily or 2–3 x per week) □ □ □

Doppler (1–2 x weekly) □ □ □

Repeat growth scan in two weeks □ □ □

12 Can happen as outpatient or inpatient □ □ □

13 Need for regular BP and urine checks □ □ □

14 Likely need for early delivery if fetal
concern □ □ □

Induction or Caesarean □ □ □

15 Need for steroids for lung maturity □ □ □

16 Neonatal prognosis very good after 34
weeks □ □ □

17 Possible neonatal complications:

RDS □ □ □

Feeding □ □ □

Hypothermia. □ □ □

18 Reassure major complications rare □ □ □

19 Explains in a clear non-jargonistic manner □ □ □

20 Invites patient's questions and answers
appropriately □ □ □

Answers

Comment

Intrauterine growth restriction is associated with pre-eclampsia, smoking, maternal drug use (eg prescribed drugs like ß-blockers or illicit drugs such as cocaine), maternal disease (eg SLE, renal diease), viral infection, eg CMV and chromosomal abnormalities. Commonly, no underlying cause is found but placental function is poor, resulting in chronic fetal hypoxia and subsequent redistribution of blood flow to the vital organs, eg brain, heart, adrenals. Consequently head measurements are often relatively normal but AC is reduced because of use of hepatic glycogen stores (asymmetrical IUGR). Reduced fetal renal perfusion leads to reduced urine output and oligohydramnios. Reduced end-diastolic flow is the result of increased downstream placental vascular resistance.

Increased fetal surveillance (kick-charts, 2–3 x weekly CTGs, Doppler 2 x weekly and 2-weekly growth scans) is vital to ensure appropriate timing of delivery. Early delivery is likely and may be either by IOL or Caesarean section. Corticosteroids are, therefore, administered to increase fetal lung maturity and try and reduce the risk of RDS. Neonatal outcome is usually excellent after 34 weeks.

STATION 2.32

Investigation

1 Crown-rump length.
2 Increased nuchal translucency.
   Chromosomal abnormality (eg Down's syndrome).
   Congenital heart disease is acceptable.
3 Chorionic villus sampling (CVS).
   Amniocentesis.
4 Ovary with polycystic morphology.
5 Obesity   Hirsuitism
   Oligo/amenorrhoea (infertility is acceptable)   Hypertension
   Type 2 DM   Hyperlipidaemia
   Acne   Menorrhagia
6 Lemon head.
7 Frontal lobe collapse secondary to spina bifida.
8 Pre-conceptual folic acid.

STATION 2.33

Instruments

1 Amnihook used for amniotomy (ARM) to either induce or augment labour.
2 Fetal scalp electrode – used when transabdominal CTG monitoring is sub-standard
   or inadequate.
3 Informed consent.
   Have an appropriate indication (eg fetal distress, maternal exhaustion).
   Fully dilated.
   Adequate analgesia.
   Empty bladder.
   Position defined.
   Adequate descent (at least to the level of the ischial spines).
   No contraindications (eg HIV, fetal bleeding disorder).
4 Maternal – vaginal, cervical, perineal trauma and haemorrhage.
   Fetal – cephalhaematoma, retinal haemorrhage, intracranial bleeding
   (rarely).
5 D – Ventouse is the instrument of choice as it has reduced maternal trauma
   compared with forceps.

Chapter 3:
Endocrine and Breast
Answers

Chapter 3

Endocrine and Breast Answers

STATION 3.1

Patient History

I am a 25-year-old engineering student, and I have been unwell for 4–5 months. Initially I had a headache in the front of my head, which has slowly worsened, particularly in the mornings. The headache radiates from the front to the top of my head. I do not get nauseated but along with the headaches I notice a loss of peripheral vision which has forced me to give up playing football and driving a car. In the last month I have had to buy larger shoes and during the recent cold spell noticed my gloves were also too small. My girlfriend has commented that 'your face seems to be widening' and I have noticed that my teeth don't seem to fit properly inside my mouth. I have not had any other symptoms of note and I am on no regular medicines other than some paracetamol for the headaches. No one in my family has any endocrine or autoimmune diseases. I am worried that something is seriously wrong. The headaches are affecting my concentration when I am studying which is also a big concern because I have finals coming up.

Assessment	Good	Adequate	Poor/not done
1 Appropriate introduction (full name and role)	☐	☐	☐
2 Explains purpose of interview	☐	☐	☐
3 Establishes reason for patient's attendance	☐	☐	☐
4 Establishes the duration of the illness	☐	☐	☐
5 Establishes the presence of local pituitary symptoms: *Headache: site, radiation, relieving/exacerbating factors*	☐	☐	☐
Visual disturbance, in particular loss of peripheral vision	☐	☐	☐

6 Establishes the presence of systemic
features of acromegaly:

Overbiting mandible/enlarged tongue ☐ ☐ ☐

Change in facial appearance ☐ ☐ ☐

7 Confirms hands/feet enlargement
Proximal limb weakness ☐ ☐ ☐

Symptoms of hyperprolactinaemia,

eg galactorrhoea ☐ ☐ ☐

Carpal tunnel symptoms ☐ ☐ ☐

Sweating; skin changes ☐ ☐ ☐

Symptoms of diabetes mellitus ☐ ☐ ☐

8 Establishes general features of endocrine
disease, eg weight changes and sleep
problems ☐ ☐ ☐

9 Excludes family history of endocrine
disease ☐ ☐ ☐

10 Elicits patient's concerns and responds
sensitively ☐ ☐ ☐

11 Appropriate questioning technique ☐ ☐ ☐

12 Avoids or explains jargon ☐ ☐ ☐

13 Summarises history back to patient,
including concerns ☐ ☐ ☐

14 Systematic, organised approach ☐ ☐ ☐

15 Makes a reasonable attempt at the
diagnosis ☐ ☐ ☐

SP to mark:

16 The student was easy to talk to ☐ ☐ ☐

Diagnosis

Growth hormone secreting pituitary tumour with local pituitary and systemic features
of acromegaly.

STATION 3.2

Patient History

I am 21 years old and I have had problems with my periods for the last 6 months. My periods began when I was 13 and they have generally been regular, lasting 4–6 days and coming every 24–27 days. My periods have now become increasingly irregular, and now last anything from 1 to 11 days and come every 33–45 days. I have never been pregnant and am not using any form of contraception. I have not had sexual intercourse for over a year as my long-term boyfriend is working in the Gulf.

I have recently noticed some milk coming out of my nipples. This is weird and I'm upset about it. I have had no headaches or visual problems. I am otherwise generally well, my weight is stable and I am on no medications. I am anxious that I will not be able to get pregnant, as my boyfriend and I want a family eventually.

Assessment	Good	Adequate	Poor/not done
1 Appropriate introduction (full name and role)	☐	☐	☐
2 Explains purpose of interview	☐	☐	☐
3 Establishes presenting problem	☐	☐	☐
4 Establishes the duration of the present illness	☐	☐	☐
5 Establishes the time of the patient's menarche	☐	☐	☐
6 Establishes her normal menstrual cycle	☐	☐	☐
7 Establishes precise history of menstrual irregularity	☐	☐	☐
8 Establishes obstetric history	☐	☐	☐
9 Establishes method of contraception, if being used	☐	☐	☐
10 Establishes history of associated galactorrhoea	☐	☐	☐
11 Excludes local pituitary symptoms, eg headache and visual disturbances	☐	☐	☐

Answers

12 Excludes other causes of menstrual
    problems:

    Pregnancy ☐ ☐

    Weight loss ☐ ☐

    Drugs ☐ ☐

    Stress ☐ ☐

    Thyroid disease ☐ ☐

13 Elicits patient's concern and responds
    sensitively ☐ ☐ ☐

14 Appropriate questioning technique ☐ ☐ ☐

15 Avoids or explains jargon ☐ ☐ ☐

16 Summarises history back to patient,
    including concerns ☐ ☐ ☐

17 Makes a reasonable attempt at the
    diagnosis ☐ ☐ ☐

18 Systematic, organised approach ☐ ☐ ☐

SP to mark

19 The doctor was empathic ☐ ☐ ☐

Diagnosis

Prolactinoma – with oligomenorrhoea and galactorrhoea.

Comment

Hyperprolactinaemia may be physiological or pathological. Physiological causes
include stimulation of the nipples (sexual or suckling), sexual intercourse, pregnancy
and stress. Pathological causes include micro and macroadenomas of the pituitary
gland, acromegaly, disorders causing interference of the hypothalamic/pituitary stalk
(eg suprasellar expansion of a pituitary tumour), polycystic ovary syndrome,
hypothyroidism, renal and hepatic failure and idiopathic. Dopaminergic antagonists
are a common cause, eg metaclopramide and the phenothiazines as well as other
medications, eg cimetidine and methyldopa. The oral contraceptives containing
oestrogens may cause it, but there is no causal link between these pills and
prolactinomas.

Prolactin release is inhibited by dopaminergic control from the hypothalamus. The treatment of pathological causes of hyperprolactinaemia is, therefore, based on dopamine agonists. Bromocriptine may be given either in tablet or pessary form and is often used as the only treatment in pituitary microadenomas. Bromocriptine has many gastrointestinal side-effects and is being superseded by other dopamine agonists, particularly cabergoline. Lisuride and pergolide are also used.

STATION 3.3

Patient History

I am a 34-year-old secretary and have previously been fit and well. Over the last 8–12 months, I have been unwell with various ailments. Initially I felt lethargic and not myself. Over the next few months I lost weight around the shoulders and hips and it all seemed to collect around my tummy. I have also developed deep purple stripes over my abdomen, which are much the same as stretch marks but ten times worse. More recently I have started having problems with hair and spots around my chin. I feel increasingly weak, particularly when standing up from a chair. In the last few weeks I have been permanently thirsty and am drinking 4–5 litres of fluid a day. I have had no headaches or visual disturbances and am otherwise relatively well, with no other specific symptoms. My mother has diabetes and a thyroid problem, as did my grandmother. I am not and never have been on any regular medications. I am very concerned about what could be wrong. I hate the other body changes and am feeling miserable about the whole thing.

Assessment	Good	Adequate	Poor/not done
1 Appropriate introduction (full name and role)	☐	☐	☐
2 Explains purpose of interview	☐	☐	☐
3 Establishes the duration of the illness	☐	☐	☐
4 Establishes weight gain, principally around the abdomen	☐	☐	☐
5 Establishes wasting and power loss around the shoulders and hips	☐	☐	☐
6 Confirms the presence of striae, bruising, acne and hirsutism	☐	☐	☐
7 Establishes symptoms of hyperglycaemia	☐	☐	☐
8 Excludes symptoms of local pituitary disease	☐	☐	☐
9 Excludes symptoms of other endocrine disease	☐	☐	☐
10 Establishes family history of endocrine disease	☐	☐	☐

11 Excludes the use of long-term steroids ☐ ☐ ☐

12 Establishes otherwise
    systemically well ☐ ☐ ☐

13 Elicits patient's concerns and responds
    sensitively ☐ ☐ ☐

14 Appropriate questioning technique ☐ ☐ ☐

15 Avoids or explains jargon ☐ ☐ ☐

16 Summarises history back to patient,
    including concerns ☐ ☐ ☐

17 Systematic, organised approach ☐ ☐ ☐

18 Makes a reasonable attempt at diagnosis ☐ ☐ ☐

Diagnosis

Cushing's disease.

STATION 3.4

Patient History

I am 18 years old and, over the last year, I have been getting increasingly irregular periods. My periods started when I was aged 12 and they were regular, with a cycle of 4–5 days every 26–28 days until the age of 16–17 when I began to put on a lot of weight. In the last year my cycle has become very irregular, lasting 1–9 days every 23–35 days. I have put on about 15 kgs in the last 18 months and have had a lot of problems with acne and hair growth around the chin and face. I feel ugly and have stopped going out with my friends. I wanted to go to college but could not face it looking like this. I do not have a boyfriend and have had no sexual contact in the last 2 years. I am not on the Pill. I am otherwise well and have had no other significant symptoms. I am not on any medications and have no family history of note.

Assessment	Good	Adequate	Poor/not done
1 Appropriate introduction (full name and role)	☐	☐	☐
2 Explains purpose of interview	☐	☐	☐
3 Establishes duration of the illness	☐	☐	☐
4 Establishes menarche and normal menstrual cycle	☐	☐	☐
5 Establishes present menstrual cycle	☐	☐	☐
6 Confirms obesity, asks about weight problems	☐	☐	☐
7 Establishes associated history of acne and hirsutism	☐	☐	☐
8 Excludes symptoms of pituitary tumour and hyperprolactinaemia	☐	☐	☐
9 Asks about general symptoms, eg loss of libido, sleep	☐	☐	☐
10 Excludes family history of endocrine disease	☐	☐	☐
11 Elicits patient's concerns and responds sensitively	☐	☐	☐
12 Appropriate questioning technique	☐	☐	☐

13 Avoids or explains jargon	☐	☐	☐
14 Summarises history back to patient, including concerns	☐	☐	☐
15 Systematic, organised approach	☐	☐	☐
16 Makes a reasonable attempt at a diagnosis	☐	☐	☐

Diagnosis

Polycystic ovary syndrome.

Comment

Polycystic ovary syndrome is a common cause of menstrual irregularity, sub-fertility, acne and hirsutism. The principal pathological features are multiple cysts of the ovaries associated with an increase in androgen production by the ovaries and adrenal glands. The initiating mechanism for these processes remains unclear.

The diagnosis is confirmed on ultasound scan of the ovaries and biochemically by the raised luteinising hormone LH: follicle stimulating hormone FSH ratio (>2:1), although the FSH level is often normal or low. Other findings include a raised total androgen level, a low sex hormone binding globulin SHBG and hyperprolactinaemia.

It is important to exclude signs of virilisation, eg clitoromegaly, as adrenal carcinomas may present in a similar fashion.

Answers

STATION 3.5

Patient History

I am 54 years old and work as a supermarket manager. I was fit and well until 4 months ago. Initially I felt unwell without any specific symptoms, just off colour and tired. More recently I have been unable to concentrate on anything, such as watching television or reading the newspaper. My work is really being affected and I'm concerned that I might lose my job.

In the last few weeks none of my clothes seem to fit and when I went to the GP, she commented that my weight had increased over 7 kgs in the last year. I am not eating any more than usual and can't understand how I've put on this amount of weight. I have been constipated recently, which is unusual for me, but I've had no other change in bowel habit. My hair seems very dry and feels terrible.

I have these patches of non-pigmented skin, which my sister and mother both have. My mother also had thyroid gland problems. I am on no medications and am otherwise well.

Assessment	Good	Adequate	Poor/not done
1 Appropriate introduction (full name and role)	☐	☐	☐
2 Explains purpose of interview	☐	☐	☐
3 Establishes the duration of the symptoms	☐	☐	☐
4 Establishes nature of 'croaky voice', eg complete loss of voice; other speech problems, eg dysphasia	☐	☐	☐
5 Excludes stridor and other upper respiratory tract symptoms, eg nasal discharge and pharyngitis	☐	☐	☐
6 Quantifies weight gain and dietary habits	☐	☐	☐
7 Establishes other symptoms of hypothyroidism:			
Cold intolerance		☐	☐
Lethargy and malaise		☐	☐
Constipation		☐	☐
Dry, coarse hair		☐	☐
Poor concentration		☐	☐

Answers

8 Establishes history of other autoimmune disease, eg pernicious anaemia, vitiligo, diabetes ☐ ☐ ☐

9 Establishes family history of autoimmune disease ☐ ☐ ☐

10 Elicits patient's concerns and responds sensitively ☐ ☐ ☐

11 Appropriate questioning technique ☐ ☐ ☐

12 Avoids or explains jargon ☐ ☐ ☐

13 Summarises history back to patient, including concerns ☐ ☐ ☐

14 Systematic, organised approach ☐ ☐ ☐

15 Summarises findings and makes a reasonable attempt at the diagnosis ☐ ☐ ☐

Answers

Diagnosis

Primary hypothyroidism with previous history of vitiligo.

Comment

Distinguishing symptoms of thyrotoxicosis

- Heat intolerance patient may feel hot and bothered, sweating
- Palpitations: may be a precipitant of atrial fibrillation. All patients presenting with atrial fibrillation should have a thyroid function test
- Diarrhoea
- Weight loss
- Tremor
- Proximal myopathy/weakness.

Graves' disease is an autoimmune disease of the thyroid which may present incidentally, with the patient being euthyroid, thyrotoxic or hypothyroid. It is characterised by Graves' eye disease, now termed Graves' orbitopathy, pre-tibial myxoedema and thyroid achropachy, which is pseudo-clubbing of the fingernails, swelling of the distal phalanges and periosteal bone formation.

STATION 3.6

Patient History

I am 54 years old and was diagnosed as having diabetes mellitus 10 years ago when I was admitted with my first myocardial infarction. Subsequently, I have had a further MI, 8 years ago, but have been well since. I test my blood with BM stix on one day in each week at 7am and then 2 hours after each meal. The readings usually show 4–7, with occasional 7–11. I stick to the diabetic diet quite strictly and take gliclazide tablets 80 mg BD. I also take Atenolol 50 mg od and aspirin 75 mg once a day. Over the last 8 years my weight has remained steady at 78 kg, after losing 16 kg in the 18 months after my initial MI. I stopped smoking after my second MI. I previously smoked 20 cigarettes per day. My lipids are normal. I do have the occasional beer but no more than 4–5 pints per week. I am otherwise well and have had no eye or foot problems. I have not had any recent angina and have had no other vascular or neurological symptoms. As far as I know my kidneys are working well. I feel pleased about my diabetic control and that I have not started smoking again or eating the wrong food.

Assessment	Good	Adequate	Poor/not done
1 Appropriate introduction (full name and role)	☐	☐	☐
2 Explains purpose of interview	☐	☐	☐
3 Establishes method, frequency and results of testing	☐	☐	☐
4 Establishes method of control and compliance	☐	☐	☐
5 Establishes weight control and dietary compliance	☐	☐	☐

6 Specifically asks about the following complications:

Macrovascular disease:

IHD, stroke, PVD ☐ ☐ ☐

Microvascular disease: ☐ ☐ ☐

retinopathy, nephropathy ☐ ☐ ☐

Neuropathic disease: sensory neuropathy ☐ ☐ ☐

Visual problems ☐ ☐ ☐

Foot problems ☐ ☐ ☐

7 Establishes/excludes associated risk factors, eg cigarettes, alcohol excess and hypercholesterolaemia ☐ ☐ ☐

8 Establishes frequency and method of follow up at outpatients and GP clinics ☐ ☐ ☐

9 Appropriate questioning technique ☐ ☐ ☐

10 Avoids or explains jargon ☐ ☐ ☐

11 Summarises history back to patient ☐ ☐ ☐

12 Summarises the case to the examiner with the correct deductions ☐ ☐ ☐

13 Systematic and organised approach ☐ ☐ ☐

SP to mark

14 The student was empathic ☐ ☐ ☐

15 The student acknowledged my efforts ☐ ☐ ☐

Answers

STATION 3.7

Patient History

I am 21 years old and work in a factory. Previously, I have been well but over the last 3 to 4 months I have become increasingly lethargic and have suffered recurrent vaginal thrush infections. I have noticed I have been drinking 4–5 bottles of diet coke a day and am forever going to pass water. In the last 3 weeks I have lost about 5 kg in weight and it was this that finally prompted me to go to the local doctor. My grandmother and an uncle on my mother's side both had diabetes and an aunt had thyroid problems. I smoke 20 cigarettes per day and drink between 20–30 units of alcohol in the form of vodka and lemonade, mainly at weekends. I do not eat a lot of sweet things and maintain my weight at 61 kg. I am 1.65 m in height. I do not do any regular exercise. I'm worried that I have diabetes because I have seen the problems it caused my grandmother.

Assessment	Good	Adequate	Poor/not done
1 Appropriate introduction (full name and role	☐	☐	☐
2 Explains purpose of interview	☐	☐	☐
3 Establishes the duration of the presenting illness	☐	☐	☐
4 Establishes history of polyuria and polydypsia	☐	☐	☐
5 Establishes history of recurrent vaginal candidiasis	☐	☐	☐
6 Establishes history of recent weight loss	☐	☐	☐
7 Establishes family history of diabetes and thyroid disease	☐	☐	☐
8 Excludes eye, foot and other complications	☐	☐	☐
9 Establishes associated risk factors – alcohol, dietary excess and smoking	☐	☐	☐
10 Elicits patient's concerns and responds sensitively	☐	☐	☐
11 Appropriate questioning technique	☐	☐	☐

12 Avoids or explains jargon	☐	☐	☐
13 Summarises history back to patient, including concerns	☐	☐	☐
14 Makes the correct diagnosis	☐	☐	☐
15 Is able to discuss future management in an appropriate manner	☐	☐	☐
16 Systematic and organised approach	☐	☐	☐

Diagnosis

Newly diagnosed insulin-dependent diabetes mellitus.

Comment

Management plan

1 Investigations: FBC, U+Es, glucose, HBA1c, lipids; urinalysis to exclude ketonuria, proteinuria and glycosuria.
2 Examination: Full examination to include ophthalmoscopy and neurological assessment.
3 Treatment: Admit to hospital and start on insulin; before discharge patient should be able administer insulin injections and have a reasonable understanding of the disease and possible complications.

Education principally from diabetic liaison nurse; reinforced by doctors, dietician assessment and education viz: dietary planning, reduce/stop smoking and alcohol excess, exercise.

Answers

STATION 3.8

Patient History

I am 21 years old and 3 days ago I have just been told, that I have diabetes mellitus. I have seen the dietician and the diabetic liaison sister, who have answered a lot of my questions. I have had a go at injecting myself with insulin but am not too confident as yet. I understand quite a lot about the disorder as my uncle is a diabetic, but he takes tablets. I would particularly like you to tell me:

- Will I always need to take insulin or may I one day be put on tablets instead?
- Will I be able to have children?
- I have heard that diabetics go blind and have strokes. Is this true?

Assessment	Good	Adequate	Poor/not done
1 Appropriate introduction (full name and role)	☐	☐	☐
2 Explains purpose of interview	☐	☐	☐
3 Establishes patient's current understanding of the disease	☐	☐	☐
4 Explains in a clear manner:			
What diabetes means	☐	☐	☐
Treatment with insulin	☐	☐	☐
Reinforcement of diet	☐	☐	☐
Blood or urine testing	☐	☐	☐
Possible complications	☐	☐	☐
Importance of compliance	☐	☐	☐
What to do for a 'hypo'	☐	☐	☐
Associated risk factors -	☐	☐	☐
Alcohol excess and smoking	☐	☐	☐
5 Gives clear explanation, avoiding or explaining jargon	☐	☐	☐

Answers

6 Invites further questions and responds
   sensitively and appropriately to patient's
   concerns   ☐   ☐   ☐

7 Checks patient's understanding of
   information   ☐   ☐   ☐

8 Systematic and organised approach   ☐   ☐   ☐

STATION 3.9

Assessment	Good	Adequate	Poor/not done
1 Appropriate introduction (full name and role)	☐	☐	☐
2 Explains examination and obtains verbal consent	☐	☐	☐
3 Observes patient, commenting on: presence/absence of any hypo/hyperthyroidism	☐	☐	☐
4 Observes & comments on neck mass from initial anterior position	☐	☐	☐
5 Asks patient to sip water and hold it in her mouth; then instructs to swallow and comments on movement of mass with swallowing	☐	☐	☐
6 Examines from behind, commenting on:			
Site	☐	☐	☐
Size	☐	☐	☐
Shape	☐	☐	☐
Surface	☐	☐	☐
Consistency	☐	☐	☐
Attachments (deep & superficial)	☐	☐	☐
Presence/absence of lymphadenopathy	☐	☐	☐

7 Repeats assessment of mass whilst
  swallowing water – while palpating
  from behind   ☐   ☐   ☐

8 Returns to front of patient and assesses
  from front:

  Thyroid bruit   ☐   ☐   ☐

  Retrosternal extension   ☐   ☐   ☐

  Transillumination   ☐   ☐   ☐

9 Treats patient courteously throughout;
  thanks patient on completion   ☐   ☐   ☐

10 Presents findings in fluent, logical manner ☐   ☐   ☐

STATION 3.10

Assessment	Good	Adequate	Poor/not done
1 Appropriate introduction (full name and role)	☐	☐	☐
2 Explains examination and obtains verbal consent	☐	☐	☐
3 Observes patient, commenting on: obvious dysthyroid signs (eg agitation, exophthalmos)	☐	☐	☐
4 Observes and comments on neck swelling from front	☐	☐	☐
5 Asks patient to sip water and hold it in her mouth; then instructs to swallow and comments on movement of mass with swallowing	☐	☐	☐
6 Examines from behind, commenting on:			
Site		☐	☐
Size		☐	☐
Shape		☐	☐
Surface		☐	☐
Consistency		☐	☐
Attachments (deep & superficial)		☐	☐
Presence/absence of lymphadenopathy		☐	☐
7 Repeats examination from behind while swallowing water	☐	☐	☐
8 Assesses from front:			
Thyroid bruit		☐	☐
Retrosternal extension		☐	☐
Transillumination		☐	☐

Answers

9   Is courteous throughout;thanks patient
    on completion   ☐   ☐   ☐

10   Presents findings in fluent, logical manner ☐   ☐   ☐

Comment

Examination of the thyroid gland is an essential skill, which is critically assessed in any clinical examination. Following inspection from the front and side, palpation for the gland and cervical nodes must be commenced from behind. A positive 'swallowing test' must be elicited, as it confirms the swelling as part of the thyroid. Protrusion of the tongue would make a thyroglossal cyst move upwards. Stigmata of thyroid disease, including hands (sweaty palms, oncholysis, acropachy), pulse (atrial fibrillation, tachycardia/bradycardia), peripheral myopathy, eye signs (exophthalmos, lid lag, lid retraction, cranial nerve palsies, chemosis) and slow-relaxing reflexes, should all be sought.

Answers

STATION 3.11

Assessment	Good	Adequate	Poor/not done
1 Appropriate introduction (full name and role)	☐	☐	☐
2 Explains examination; obtains verbal consent	☐	☐	☐
3 Observes and comments on:			
General appearance (agitated, asthenic)			
Dysthyroid signs (eyes, tremor)	☐	☐	☐
4 Examines hands, commenting on:			
Warmth/coolness		☐	☐
Fine tremor		☐	☐
Palmar erythema		☐	☐
Onycholysis	☐	☐	☐
5 Examines radial pulse with comments	☐	☐	☐
6 Examines for proximal myopathy		☐	☐
7 Examines for eye signs and lid lag	☐	☐	☐
8 Examines for bruit over goitre		☐	☐
9 Examines for slow-relaxing reflexes	☐	☐	☐
10 Comments on features of Graves' triad if present	☐	☐	☐
11 Courteous manner and thanks patient on completion	☐	☐	☐
12 Presents findings in fluent logical manner	☐	☐	☐
13 Correctly diagnoses thyroid status clinically	☐	☐	☐

STATION 3.12

1 Fig 3.12a: Graves' disease (hyperthyroidism with exophthalmos)

   Fig 3.12b: Follicular carcinoma of thyroid with skull metastases

2 Radioisotope I^{131} scintiscan

3 Fig 3.12a:Exophthalmos-producing substance: a neuroendocrine transmitter secreted in the hypothalamus

   Fig 3.12b: A deposit of follicular carcinoma in the skull from a primary tumour of the thyroid gland

4 Fig 3.12b: Graves' disease: medical control with antithyroid agents with/without subtotal thyroidectomy

   Fig 3.12b: Follicular carcinoma of thyroid: total thyroidectomy with radio-iodine ablation of metastases.

Comment

In Graves' disease, hyperthyroidism is a result of to IgG microsomal antibodies against TSH receptors on the thyroid follicular cell, stimulating thyroid hormone production and goitre formation. Long-acting thyroid stimulating antibodies are also present, but their role is uncertain.

In follicular carcinoma of the thyroid, blood-borne spread occurs early, and total thyroidectomy, even in the absence of goitre, enables tumour deposits to be targeted by radioiodine therapy.

STATION 3.13

1 (a) **False**   (b) **False**   (c) **True**   (d) **False**   (e) **False**
This figure shows evidence of background diabetic retinopathy with blot and dot haemorrhages concentrated in the temporal quadrants. The nasal quadrants are relatively disease-free, and the macula and optic disc are normal. These changes mark the onset of microvascular complications and are often associated with early renal damage, characterised by microalbuminuria. Papilloedema is not associated with background retinopathy and remains a sinister sign for which an underlying cause should be sought.

2 (a) **True**   (b) **False**   (c) **False**   (d) **True**   (e) **False**
This figure shows background diabetic retinopathy with added maculopathy. There are blot and dot haemorrhages and several areas of hard exudate, including the areas surrounding the macula. Hard exudates have well-defined margins and represent lipid deposition within the retina.

3 (a) **True**   (b) **True**   (c) **False**   (d) **True**   (e) **False**
This slide shows evidence of extensive retinal haemorrhage with exudates. There is also a 'long boat', subhyaloid (pre-retinal) haemorrhage and a macular 'star', formed by the exudates encircling the macular. This represents severe pre-proliferative diabetic retinopathy and maculopathy.

4 (a) **True**   (b) **True**   (c) **True**   (d) **False**   (e) **False**
This slide shows pre-proliferative diabetic retinopathy with blot and dot haemorrhages soft and hard exudates. Soft exudates (cottonwool spots) have ill-defined, 'fluffy', margins as seen in the inferior temporal and upper nasal quadrants. They represent areas of impending ischaemic damage to the retina. The patient requires strict glycaemic control through diet and medication, which may be oral hypoglycaemics rather than insulin.

5 (a) **True**   (B) **True**   (c) **True**   (d) **False**   (e) **False**
This slide shows proliferative diabetic retinopathy, characterised by new vessel formation, neo-vascularisation. This is an attempt by the retina to overcome increasing ischaemia. Neovascularisation, worsening visual acuity, maculopathy and visual loss are all indications for referral to an ophthalmologist.

STATION 3.14

1 (c)

Long-term steroid use causes suppression of endogenous steroid production and is the commonest cause of Addison's disease. Patients typically present with non-specific symptoms but may present in coma. In any patient who presents with coma and hyponatraemia, Addison's should always be considered and, if no obvious cause can be attributed, the patient should be given 100 to 200 mg of IV hydrocortisone 4 to 6 hourly for 24 hours, depending on the clinical response.

2 (d)

Hypothyroidism may cause hyponatraemia associated with a macrocytosis. The hyponatraemia is secondary to increased ADH secretion and reduced free water clearance. The macrocytosis may be secondary to the thyroid disease or to associated pernicious anaemia.

3 (e)

Atypical pneumonias, eg mycoplasma, are a common cause of the syndrome of inappropiate ADH. Other causes include:

Intracerebral
Head injury
Meningitis
Encephalitis
Benign and malignant tumours
Pulmonary
Pneumonia
Tuberculosis
Small cell
Tumours
Abscess
Malignancies
Thymoma
Prostatic
Pancreatic
Lymphoma
Drugs
Chemotherapeutic agents
Chlorpropamide
Carbamazepine
Clofibrate

4 **(a)**

Psychogenic polydypsia is an uncommon cause of hyponatraemia. It is important to exclude diabetes mellitus and insipidus which may also present with polyuria. Patients with psychogenic polydypsia have a hyponatraemia associated with a low-serum osmolality and an appropiately low-urine osmolality. The diagnosis is confirmed using a water deprivation test.

5 **(b)**

The commonest cause of hyponatraemia in the older patient is the use of diuretics. Other side-effects of loop diuretics include: hypokalaemia, hypomagnesaemia and pre-renal impairment, causing a rise in urea and creatinine. Selective seratonin receptive inhibitors (SSRIs) also commonly cause hyponatraemia in the elderly.

Answers

STATION 3.15

Hypokalaemia	Hyperkalaemia
Cushing's disease	Addison's disease
Frusemide infusion	Spironolactone
Type I RTA	Type IV RTA
Fanconi's syndrome	Acute renal failure
Ectopic ACTH	Lisinopril
Conn's syndrome	
Cardiac failure with secondary hyperaldosteronism	

Comment

Cushing's disease (pituitary dependent) and Cushing's syndrome, eg ectopic ACTH secretion, cause hypokalaemia. Ectopic ACTH secretion may cause a severe hypokalaemia associated with a metabolic alkalosis. It usually arises in association with a malignant tumour, most commonly a small cell carcinoma of the lung. Addison's disease causes a hyperkalaemia and hyponatraemia with an associated metabolic acidosis.

Loop and thiazide diuretics cause hypokalaemia, whereas spironolactone and lisinopril cause potassium retention. Loop diuretics are often given in combination with amiloride to maintain normokalaemia. Lisinopril is one of the new generation of angiotension-converting enzyme (ACE) inhibitors. They cause potassium retention through their effects on the renin-angiotensin system.

Conn's syndrome (primary hyperaldosteronism) and secondary hyperaldosteronism cause hypokalaemia and a metabolic alkalosis. Secondary hyperaldosteronism arises in oedematous states, eg cardiac, renal and hepatic failure.

Type I RTA and the Fanconi's syndrome (associated with Type II RTA) cause hypokalaemia, whereas Type IV RTA causes hyperkalaemia.

STATION 3.16

Patient A:
Plasma osmolality = 2[158 + 4.9] +34+50 = 409.8
Anion gap = [158+4.9] – [12+ 102] = 48.9

The high anion gap is due to the very high lactate level. The patient's urinalysis
suggests that she is suffering from a UTI.

Diagnosis
UTI sepsis leading to lactic acidosis and hyperglycaemic coma.

Patient B:
Plasma osmolality = 2[145 + 4] +14 + 45.3 = 357.3
Anion gap = [145 + 4] – [8 + 106] = 35

The high anion gap can not be accounted for by the slightly raised lactate level. This
patient's urinalysis suggests 'heavy' ketonuria in keeping with diabetic ketoacidosis
(DKA).

Diagnosis
Pneumonia leading to diabetic ketoacidosis

Patient C
Plasma osmolality = 2[155 + 4.5] + 19 + 80 = 418
Anion Gap = [155 + 4.5] – [25 + 110] = 24.5

The slightly elevated anion gap arises from the raised lactate level which may be a
result of tissue hypoxia in severe sepsis. However compared to the other cases this
patient has a relatively normal anion gap and, as shown by his plasma osmolality,
has a hyperosmolar, non-ketotic coma (HONK).

Diagnosis
Hyperosmolar, non-ketotic hyperglycaemic coma.

Comment
If a diabetic patient is found unconscious in the street, you should always attempt to
give them some glucose. After following the basic resuscitation rules of ABC, the
easiest method is to dissolve a sachet of sugar or some honey under their tongue.
(Attempting to force sweet drinks into a semi or unconscious patient may lead to
aspiration.)

Answers

STATION 3.17

A **3 Primary hypothyroidism**

The data indicates an extremely elevated TSH with low levels of T3 and T4. Common causes include: autoimmune-disease, including Hashimoto's disease, post-thyroidectomy, irradiation and radioactive iodine therapy for thyrotoxicosis and, in mountainous regions, iodine deficiency.

B **1 Thyrotoxicosis**

The data shows a surpressed TSH level, with a raised T3 and extremely raised T4. This is the most common biochemical presentation of thyrotoxicosis. Causes of thyrotoxicosis include: autoimmune thyrotoxicosis, benign and malignant thyroid masses, multinodular goitre and acute thyroiditis.

C **5 Sick euthyroid syndrome**

In acute illness, particularly severe systemic disease, abnormal production and binding of thyroid hormones and transport proteins lead to biochemical results which do not tally. In this case, the data initially suggests the patient may have hypothyroidism, with low T3 and T4. However, the TSH is low which suggests either hypothalamic/pituitary failure or the sick euthyroid syndrome. In moderate illnesses the free T4 may be raised with a normal or raised TSH.

D **2 T3 thyrotoxicosis**

This is an uncommon cause of thyrotoxicosis. The patient has clinical symptoms and signs of thyrotoxicosis but has a T4 in the normal range. The T3, as in this case, is elevated.

E **4 Euthyroid** – The patient has normal T3, T4 and TSH.

STATION 3.18

1 (E) (f)

This woman has symptoms consistent with osteomalacia, ie proximal muscle weakness and pain. In childhood the lack of vitamin D and its metabolites lead to bony deformity, particularly of the lower limb bones, leading to the classical appearance of rickets. The bony abnormality arises as a result of ineffective osteoid mineralisation.

2 (F) (e)

This is a classic history for sarcoidosis. Black American women, particularly in the southern states of the USA have a very high incidence of the disorder. Sarcoid causes a hypercalcaemia and hypercalciuria, leading to renal tract calcification and stones.

3 (D) (a)

The premature menopause suggests long-term oestrogen deficiency, a primary risk factor for the development of osteoporosis. The disorder per se does not affect calcium levels and a raised calcium should make the physician think of associated malignancy, particularly myeloma, which may present in a similar fashion.

4 (A) (c)

This is a classic history of Paget's disease of the bone. The calcium and phosphate are unchanged by the disorder but the alkaline phosphatase is often greatly raised. This reflects the excessive bony turnover and increased osteoclastic activity. Complications of the disease include: bony pain, pathological fractures, the classic anterior bowing of the tibia, cranial nerve compression, high-output cardiac failure and rarely, osteosarcoma formation.

5 (C) (b)

Multiple myeloma is one of the commonest causes of hypercalcaemia in the elderly. Clinically it presents with bone pain. As well as hypercalcaemia, the patient has a raised ESR, often over 100, and a normochromic, normocytic anaemia. Other markers include the presence of a paraprotein in the serum, shown by plasma electrophoresis, and Bence–Jones proteins in the urine. Lytic lesions are present radiologically.

6 (B) (d)

Pseudohypoparathyroidism is a rare disorder due to end-organ resistance to the effects of parathyroid hormone. The patients are dysmorphic, with a low IQ, and shortened 4th and 5th metacarpals. Biochemically the patient appears to have hypoparathyroidism, but parathyroid levels are normal. Pseudo-pseudohypoparathyroidism is the disorder of abnormal phenotype with normal calcium metabolism.

STATION 3.19

Patient A: Cranial diabetes insipidus.

The data shows this patient to have a relatively high plasma osmolality with an inappropiately low-urinary osmolality. During the 8 hours of water deprivation the urinary osmolality remains very low, implying an inability to concentrate the urine, ie no effective ADH. However, when the patient is given DDAVP, an ADH analogue, the urine concentrates, with a fall in plasma osmolality. This implies the renal tubules do have the capacity to react to ADH, ie the posterior pituitary is failing to secrete ADH appropriately. If the data had been unaffected by the ADH this would imply nephrogenic diabetes insipidus, where there is an insensitivity of the tubules to appropriate levels of ADH.

During a water deprivation test the patient's urine output and body weight are closely monitored. If the patient loses more than 3% of their initial body weight, the test is immediately stopped and the diagnosis of diabetes insipidus is assumed.

Patient B: Normal control.

The data is all within normal limits and is unenhanced with the addition of extra ADH. The patient concentrates urine appropriately in an attempt to conserve water in the face of a prolonged period of water deprivation.

Patient C: Psychogenic polydypsia.

Patients with this disorder present with polydypsia, polyuria and a normal plasma glucose. They are thought to have a psychiatric condition and are therefore often difficult to assess. A water deprivation test is used to exclude diabetes insipidus, although partial ADH insensitivity is difficult to differentiate. Normally, they have a low, or low normal, plasma osmolality with appropiately low-urinary osmolality. Subjected to a prolonged period of water deprivation, they will appropriately conserve water in response to ADH secretion and will thus raise their urinary osmolality. The effect of additional ADH is similar to the normal control.

STATION 3.20

1 (a) **False**   (b) **False**   (c) **True**   (d) **False**   (e) **True**

This SXR shows an enlarged pituitary fossa (Fig 3.20a). The diagnosis may be made in 70–80% of cases of acromegaly. The classic double floor of the fossa should only be diagnosed when the clinoid processes are aligned. Other SXR changes that may be seen in this condition are an enlarged, protruding mandible (prognathism), which can be seen in this patient and increased interdental separation in the AP view.

2 (a) **False**   (b) **True**   (c) **False**   (d) **True**   (e) **False**

This is an AP foot radiograph of a diabetic patient showing evidence of swelling and possible gas in soft tissues, particularly over the right 2nd toe. There is also destruction of the proximal phalanx of the 2nd toe due to osteomyelitis. Note the vascular calcification which is a common sign in diabetes mellitus. Other radiological changes that may occur include Charcot (neuropathic) joints and digital amputation.

3 (a) **True**   (b) **False**   (c) **True**   (d) **True**   (e) **True**

This lateral skull radiograph shows gross Paget's disease of the bone. It is important to add 'of the bone' as Paget described disorders of the nipple and scrotum as well. The radiograph shows evidence of platybasia, an invagination of the foramen magnum and skull base caused by the remodelling. This produces pressure on the upper cervical cord, medulla and lower cranial nerves and may be responsible for the neural deafness.

Four sites are classically affected: the skull, the pelvis, the tibia (sabre tibia) and other weight bearing bones. Bony abnormalities include: local warmth of the bones due to increased vascularity, pain, fractures and rarely osteosarcomatous change. Other complications include optic atrophy the result of compression of the optic nerve and high-output cardiac failure.

Answers

STATION 3.21

1 (a) **False**   (b) **False**   (c) **False**   (d) **False**   (e) **True**

This is an AP view of the pelvis and hip joints showing multiple Looser's zones of osteomalacia(indicated by arrows in fig 3.21a). The bones are of normal radiodensity. With such florid bone changes a patient would be expected to have a low-serum calcium and raised alkaline phosphatase.

2 (a) **True**   (b) **True**   (c) **True**   (d) **False**   (e) **True**

This AP thoracic inlet view of the chest shows soft tissue swelling and calcification on the right side of the neck consistent with a calcified thyroid nodular goitre. The trachea is deviated to the left. Further investigations should include an autoantibody screen, thyroid function tests, fine needle aspirate (FNA) and radioisotope scan of the thyroid.

3 (a) **True**   (b) **True**   (c) **True**   (d) **False**   (e) **True**

This is an AP chest radiograph of a baby showing the 'sail' sign of a prominent thymus gland.

STATION 3.22

1 This is a radioisotope scan of the thyroid gland showing a 'toxic' or hot nodule in the right thyroid lobe with suppression of the rest of the gland. This most likely represents a solitary benign active nodule or may represent part of a multinodular goitre. Inactive or cold nodules represent areas of fibrosis, cysts or in 10% of cases a malignant tumour.

2 This is a pancreatic angiogram, the arrows defining the margins of a mass, which is most likely to be an insulinoma. Insulinomas are often very small tumours and may be difficult to define with other forms of imaging such as CT or MRI scan.

3 This is a CT scan taken through the orbits. The structures are:
   (A) Thickened right medial rectus
   (B) Right optic nerve
   (C) Right lateral rectus
   (D) Proptosed right eye

The scan shows a proptosed right eye with a greatly thickened right medial rectus, (compare the left and right sides).These abnormalities are consistent with Graves' orbitopathy. Graves' thyroid disease is an autoimmune disease which may cause the patient to be hypo-, eu- or hyperthyroid. The classic triad of the disorder is thyroid achropathy, orbitopathy and pre-tibial myxoedema. Patients should have TFTs and thyroid autoantibodies and a general autoantibody screen.

Answers

STATION 3.23

1 AP view of the thoracic inlet shows marked displacement of the trachea to the right by a large goitre that extends to just below the sternal notch.
2 Thyroid enlargement (goitre) extending to below the thoracic inlet.
3 Lateral views of the neck and thoracic inlet chest radiograph.
4 Surgical removal of the goitre (a subtotal or total thyroidectomy).

Comment
Retrosternal goitres are uncommon and may compress the trachea, oesophagus and the jugular veins at the thoracic inlet. Emergency surgical decompression is rarely indicated, and thyroid and respiratory function must be assessed during work-up for thyroidectomy.

STATION 3.24

(A) Cerebral cortex
(B) Genu of corpus callosum
(C) Suprasellar tumour extension
(D) Pituitary fossa and tumour
(E) Sphenoidal air sinus
(F) Collicular plate
(G) Fourth ventricle
(H) Cerebellar cortex

STATION 3.25

(A) Liver
(B) Adrenal adenoma
(C) Aorta
(D) Vertebral body
(E) Left crus of diagphragm
(F) Upper pole of left kidney
(G) Spleen
(H) Stomach with contrast and air bubble above fluid level

STATION 3.26

1 Radioisotope scan of the thyroid gland.
   Radioactive iodine (I^{131} or I^{123}) or technitium (Tc^{99m}).
2 Lower pole of left lobe contains a circumscribed lesion that does not take up the radioisotope – a cold spot:
   > A thyroid cyst.
   > An area of haemorrhage.
   > A thyroid adenoma.
   > A thyroid carcinoma.
3 Ultrasound scan of the thyroid to determine if the lesion is solid or cystic and enable a guided fine needle aspiration biopsy of the lesion. (The incidence of thyroid cancer in a solitary solid nodule is 12%.)

Comment
A 'hot' nodule with its increased uptake of radio-iodine is usually diagnostic of a hyperactive nodule, but occasionally a focus of follicular carcinoma may appear likewise. A thyroid cyst, which also appears as a 'cold' nodule on scintiscanning is readily distinguished on ultrasound scanning. Fine needle aspiration cytology is useful in confirming anaplastic tumours and bony metastatic deposits of follicular tumours.

Answers

STATION 3.27

Patient History

I am a 48-year-old solicitor and have recently developed symptoms of the menopause. My last normal period was over 7 months ago, although I have had three or four further scanty bleeds since. I have flushing, irritability and more recently dyspareunia secondary to vaginal dryness. I understand from magazines about the treatment and would like to start. I am a non-smoker and a keen walker. I am otherwise well and have had no serious illness in the past. My last smear was 4 years ago and was normal.

The questions I would like answered are:

How long will I be on the treatment?

Does it have any side-effects?

Will it increase my risk of cancer?

Assessment	Good	Adequate	Poor/not done
1 Appropriate introduction (full name and role)	☐	☐	☐
2 Establishes reason for visit	☐	☐	☐
3 Establishes patient's last period and menopausal symptoms	☐	☐	☐
4 Establishes patient's understanding of the treatment	☐	☐	☐
5 Discusses the treatment specifically mentioning:			
Protection against osteoporosis	☐	☐	☐
Possible protection against IHD	☐	☐	☐
Stops symptoms of oestrogen deficiency	☐	☐	☐
Small risk of thrombo-embolic disease	☐	☐	☐
Many treatments still cause cyclical blood loss	☐	☐	☐
Recommended treatment is for about 5 years	☐	☐	☐

6 Establishes whether patient has had any
   gynaecological or breast malignancies   ☐   ☐   ☐

7 Establishes other risk factors
   for osteoporosis   ☐   ☐   ☐

8 Gives clear explanation, avoiding or
   explaining jargon   ☐   ☐   ☐

9 Answers the patient's questions in a
   reasonable manner   ☐   ☐   ☐

10 Checks patient's understanding of
   information   ☐   ☐   ☐

11 Systematic and organised approach   ☐   ☐   ☐

Comment

Over the last 10 years hormone replacement therapy for post-menopausal women has become both accepted and demanded by women. It has few contraindications and although there are no long-term studies on its effects, the short-term therapy recommended at present seems to have major advantages and few disadvantages.

Treatment is recommended to post-menopausal women for about 5 years. A definitive time period is as yet unknown. Therapy alleviates symptoms of oestrogen deficiency such as flushing and vaginal atrophy; delays the onset of bone loss, leading to osteoporosis; and increases HDL and decreases LDL levels.

There is an increased risk of thrombo-embolic disease but this is much smaller than that associated with the oral contraceptive pill, and should be viewed in relation to other risks, such as smoking, previous thrombo-embolic events and obesity. Caution is also recommended in patients with previous breast and gynaecological malignancies, although there is no definitive evidence that HRT causes an increase in these cancers. Newer treatments with continuous therapy have meant that withdrawal vaginal bleeding does not occur. This makes it a more attractive prospect, particularly in elderly women who have not had periods for many years.

Answers

STATION 3.28

Answers and explanations

1 (C) (b)

Actrapid, as its name suggests, is a short-acting insulin. It is used in qds insulin treatments as the pre-prandial insulin. It is also commonly used intravenously with an insulin sliding scale. Insulin is principally manufactured by genetic engineering and, therefore, allergic reaction is rare. Local infection may occur at injection sites and lipoatrophy may also occur if the sites are not routinely rotated.

2 (E) (d)

Metformin is the only biguanide used today, as its sister molecule, Phenformin, caused severe lactic acidosis. Metformin may also produce this side-effect and must be used with caution in patients with unstable angina, hepatic and renal impairment, as all these predispose to increased levels of the drug and acidosis.

3 (A) (e)

Tolbutamide is a short-acting sulphonylurea with a half-life of 6–8 hours. The main side-effect of this group is hypoglycaemia and patients must be pre-warned about hypoglycaemic symptoms.

4 (B) (a)

Acarbose is an a glucosidase inhibitor which is principally used as an adjuvnt therapy in NIDDM. The drug inhibits amylase, maltase and sucrase, thus decreasing carbohydrate absorption and reducing post-prandial hyperglycaemia. The side-effects of flatulence and bloating limit its use.

5 (D) (c)

Chlorpropamide is a long-acting sulphonylurea. It may cause SIADH, which was previously utilised in patients with diabetes insipidus and flushing with alcohol, although this is rare. Glibenclamide and chlorpropamide should not be used in the elderly as their long half-life and patients' renal impairment lead to increased risk of hypoglycaemia.

STATION 3.29

Patient History

I am 23 years old and work as a secretary. I was admitted to hospital 4 days ago with newly diagnosed diabetes mellitus. I have been seen by the dietician and the diabetic liaison sister, who has explained the principles of insulin therapy to me. I have not as yet attempted to inject myself. The nurses have been showing me how to draw up the insulin and where and how to give the injections. I am feeling positive and want to get on top of this disease.

Assessment	Good	Adequate	Poor/not done
1 Appropriate introduction (full name and role)	☐	☐	☐
2 Explains purpose of interview	☐	☐	☐
3 Establishes the patient's understanding of the treatment	☐	☐	☐
4 Explains the following: *Establishes patient has correct equipment*	☐	☐	☐
Checks using correct insulin which is in date	☐	☐	☐
Uses clean syringe and needle for each injection	☐	☐	☐
Inverts the insulin and draws it up to the correct units required	☐	☐	☐
Cleans the injection site using an antiseptic wipe	☐	☐	☐
Forms a pinch of skin and injects through it at 90 degrees	☐	☐	☐
5 Establishes patient has understood by getting her to demonstrate the procedure	☐	☐	☐
6 Invites patient's questions and answers in an appropriate manner	☐	☐	☐
7 Stresses the importance of rotating injection sites between the abdomen, thighs and buttocks	☐	☐	☐

Answers

Never missing doses of insulin: ☐ ☐ ☐

*To seek medical attention if unable to
take insulin or if unable to eat after
insulin* ☐ ☐ ☐

*Tight glycaemic control leads to fewer
complications* ☐ ☐ ☐

*Insulin should be administered
approximately 30 minutes prior
to a meal* ☐ ☐ ☐

8 Clear explanation, avoiding or
explaining jargon ☐ ☐ ☐

9 Checks patient's understanding of
explanation ☐ ☐ ☐

10 Systematic and organised approach ☐ ☐ ☐

STATION 3.30a

Patient History

I am a 19 years old nurse and recently underwent surgery for a pituitary tumour. I have had some of my new medicines explained to me by the consultant but have not really understood all the treatments.

I would like to know the answers to the following questions:

(a) Will I be able to get pregnant on these hormones?
(b) Will I get big muscles with these steroid tablets?
(c) Is it true that I will probably have to take these tablets for life?

Assessment	Good	Adequate	Poor/not done
1 Appropriate introduction (full name and role)	☐	☐	☐
2 Explains purpose of interview	☐	☐	☐
3 Establishes patient's current understanding of her treatment	☐	☐	☐
4 Explains the following: *How the pituitary gland normally functions The drugs being used are to replace*	☐	☐	☐
naturally occurring hormones and will take over their function	☐	☐	☐
It is essential she never misses doses of the drugs, particularly the hydrocortisone	☐	☐	☐
5 Ensures the patient has been issued with a blue steriod card and has a medi-alert bracelet	☐	☐	☐
6 If unwell needs to seek medical advice immediately	☐	☐	☐
7 Gives information in manageable chunks	☐	☐	☐
8 Gives clear, jargon-free explanation	☐	☐	☐
9 Invites patient's questions and answers appropriately	☐	☐	☐

Answers

10 Checks what patient has understood of the information	☐	☐	☐
11 Systematic and organised approach	☐	☐	☐

Answers to Specific Questions

The removal of cyclical FSH/LH means it is very difficult for the patient to become pregnant. Although the FSH/LH replacement restores oestrogen activity essential for cardiovascular and bone protection, it can not, under normal circumstances, reproduce a normal menstrual cycle. However, with ovulation and egg harvesting, for in vitro fertilisation and implantation, a pregnancy may be carried to term under endocrine therapy.

No. The hydrocortisone replaces only the naturally occurring steroids of the body and should not cause any side-effects, but in excess may lead to problems. It is, therefore, essential to have assessment of hormone replacement at least annually.

Yes. The hydrocortisone and thyroxine will be lifelong, but the FSH/LH are principally needed to maintain normal menstrual/ovulatory function and may be withdrawn to induce a natural menopause.

STATION 3.31

Patient History

I have been having severe pain and swelling of both breasts: the left breast more so than the right for the past 8 months. The pain is relieved during periods but gradually builds up afterwards. My breasts feel tender and lumpy, and I find it uncomfortable to lie on my side. I am finding it difficult to do my housework, particularly carrying the shopping and coping with my 3-year-old toddler. I have two other children, all of whom were breastfed.

My breasts have not bothered me in the past, and I have been well all my life. I smoke about 4 or 5 cigarettes a day, and I like drinking coffee and drink alcohol only on social occasions.

My doctor gave me pain killers and water tablets, which have not been of much help. Two weeks ago, I started taking evening primrose oil tablets, which were recommended by a friend who had the same problem; it has not had any effect. I am worried that this could be something serious. Also the pain makes me irritable, especially with the children.

Assessment	Good	Adequate	Poor/not done
1 Appropriate introduction (full name and role)	☐	☐	☐
2 Explains purpose of interview	☐	☐	☐
3 Establishes site, duration and periodicity of presenting symptoms	☐	☐	☐
4 Asks about other breast symptoms; past history of breast disease	☐	☐	☐
5 Establishes current treatment (if any)	☐	☐	☐
6 Asks about menstrual cycle, contraceptive use	☐	☐	☐
7 Establishes history of pregnancies, lactation, family history of breast disease	☐	☐	☐
8 Social and/or professional status; smoking habits	☐	☐	☐
9 Elicits patient's concerns and responds sensitively	☐	☐	☐

Answers

10 Appropriate questioning technique	☐	☐	☐
11 Avoids or explains jargon	☐	☐	☐
12 Summarises history back to patient, including concerns	☐	☐	☐
13 Makes a reasonable attempt at the diagnosis	☐	☐	☐
14 Systematic, organised approach	☐	☐	☐

Diagnosis
Mastalgia.

Comment
Mastalgia is cyclical breast pain and is benign. It is associated with fibroadenosis or benign breast change. Fluid retention also causes breast pain. (The contraceptive pill and smoking are aggravating factors, and coffee consumption has been implicated.) Breast support during the day and at night if necessary, with an oral diuretic, may be sufficient as an initial measure. For persisting symptoms evening primrose oil or starflower oil may be prescribed. Danazol may be tried if the above measures fail to give relief.

STATION 3.32

Patient History

I am single, aged 26, and work as a medical secretary. I am in good health and have had no trouble with my breasts, except for cyclical discomfort and swelling. I am currently not on the pill, and my periods are regular. My mother had breast cancer at the age of 38 and had a mastectomy. She is on long-term tamoxifen and is keeping well. My aunt (my mother's elder sister) developed breast cancer at the age of 52, and my cousin also had breast cancer when she was 40. They both underwent surgery and chemotherapy. I am very frightened of developing breast cancer but often feel it is inevitable.

Assessment	Good	Adequate	Poor/not done
1 Appropriate introduction (full name and role)	☐	☐	☐
2 Explains purpose of interview	☐	☐	☐
3 Establishes the presenting anxiety	☐	☐	☐
4 Establishes/excludes family history of cancer	☐	☐	☐
5 Establishes/excludes previous breast disease in patient	☐	☐	☐
6 Establishes menstrual history, pregnancy and lactation	☐	☐	☐
7 Establishes contraception/hormone therapy	☐	☐	☐
8 Social and professional history	☐	☐	☐
9 Elicits patient's concerns and responds sensitively	☐	☐	☐
10 Appropriate questioning technique	☐	☐	☐
11 Avoids or explains jargon	☐	☐	☐
12 Summarises history back to patient, including concerns	☐	☐	☐

Answers

| 13 Systematic, organised approach | ☐ | ☐ | ☐ |

SP to mark

| 14 This student was empathic | ☐ | ☐ | ☐ |

Comment

Only 1–2% of breast cancers are hereditary, and are transmitted through the breast cancer susceptibility genes (BRCA) 1 and BRCA 2 oncogenes. These genes also transmit ovarian cancer. Hereditary breast cancer usually manifests itself before the fifth decade of life. Genetic counselling is advised if two or more first-degree relatives had developed breast cancer before the age of 50 years. Genetic testing identifies the oncogene and, if it is present, the patient would require counselling with regard to close surveillance and periodic mammography. Prophylactic bilateral subcutaneous mastectomies, with prosthetic reconstruction as a means of eliminating the risk, should also be discussed.

STATION 3.33

TRUE: 1, 2a, 2b, 2c, 3a, 3b.

FALSE: 2d, 3c.

Comment

Rarely are breasts identically symmetrical in women. When one or both breasts are hypoplastic or rudimentary, breast augmentation is performed by expandable silicone implants. Hypertrophy of the breast is more common and may be corrected by reduction mammoplasty; nipple transfer and re-implantation precludes subsequent lactation.

STATION 3.34

Assessment	Good	Adequate	Poor/not done
1 Appropriate introduction (full name and role)	☐	☐	☐
2 Explains examination & obtains verbal consent	☐	☐	☐
3 Inspects patient undressed to waist, sitting up with:			
Hands by the side		☐	☐
Hands raised over head		☐	☐
Asks patient to place hands on hips and to press in	☐	☐	☐
4 Comments on breast symmetry, scars, deformities or skin changes	☐	☐	☐
5 Requests patient to lie supine at 45°:			
Palpates breast by each quadrant	☐	☐	☐
Palpates supraclavicular fossa and axilla.	☐	☐	☐
6 Comments on:			
Nipple areolar complex	☐	☐	☐
Breast quadrants	☐	☐	☐
Lymphatic drainage sites.	☐	☐	☐
7 Observes for signs of discomfort/pain while examining	☐	☐	☐
8 Palpates contralateral breast and drainage sites	☐	☐	☐
9 Palpates abdomen, commenting on the liver	☐	☐	☐
10 Concludes examination by thanking patient (requests her to dress)	☐	☐	☐
11 Presents findings in fluent, orderly manner and gives a clinical diagnosis	☐	☐	☐

Answers

Comment

Breast examination begins with inspection of the breasts with the patient seated facing the examiner. The patient is asked to place her hands on her lap, raise her hands over the head and then to place her hands on her hips and to press in. Any deformity of the breast, irregularity of its contour, skin or muscle tethering would be observed.

Palpation of the breasts is best performed in the supine, semi-recumbent position with her hands by the side and then with the hands raised over her head.

1 Observation

Face the sitting patient and observe breast symmetry, nipple orientation and skin texture, with patient relaxed and with pectoral muscles under contraction. Breast swelling or indentation may be obvious when viewed from the side or above.

2 Palpation – breast

Mastalgia is a common symptom and breast tenderness must be elicited with care and gentleness.

Findings on examination are given a P (palpation) value (P1- normal, P2- obviously benign, P3- equivocal/borderline, P4- suspicious of malignancy, P5- obviously malignant). A P3 value or higher requires further evaluation with imaging and needle biopsies.

3 Palpation – axilla

Each axillary group of lymph nodes (apical, medial, lateral, posterior and pectoral) must be palpated and commented upon.

STATION 3.35

(A) Fig 3.35a: radioisotope bone scan

Fig 3.35b: liver ultrasound scan

Fig 3.35a: uptake of isotope by the skeleton: left femur and pelvis.

Fig 3.35b: discrete hypoecogenic deposits (three in number) in the right lobe of the liver.

(B) Metastatic deposits are present in the bone and liver from the breast cancer.

(C) Local excision or radiotherapy of the primary tumour if large or prone to local complications.

Distal spread may be controlled by adjuvant chemotherapy and/or tamoxifen therapy.

Comment

Recurrent breast carcinomas must be staged, before adjuvant treatment is planned, with liver and bone scans. Local control of the recurrence is by surgical excision or radiotherapy to the chest wall. Control of systemic disease is by chemo or endocrine therapy.

STATION 3.36

Answers

1 Mammograms.

2 Both investigations show focal radiological opacity, with discrete microcalcification and distortion of the surrounding breast tissue.

3 Breast carcinomas.

4 Wire-guided excisional biopsy.

5 The patient (in the presence of a relative and/or breast nurse counsellor) is informed of the mammographic findings and the need to remove the lesion shown by means of a wire-guided biopsy for pathological examination. Confirmation of the presence of a tumour would lead to planning appropriate treatment.

Comment

Deposits of calcium in breast tissue may be in the form of macro or microcalcification. The former are large calcium deposits, which are associated with benign change. Microcalcification, however, is linked to malignancy and, when present within a mass lesion, is suggestive of cancer.

STATION 3.37

Assessment	Good	Adequate	Poor/not done
1 Palpation of the marked lesion. Cleanse skin	☐	☐	☐
2 Introduction of needle into lesion and withdrawal of plunger during repeated passes into lesion	☐	☐	☐
3 Covers puncture site with dressing	☐	☐	☐
4 Examines syringe contents Prepares smears (air-dried and in fixative). Empties remaining aspirate into container with fixative for cytospin smears	☐	☐	☐

Comment

Fine needle aspiration cytology is one of the diagnostic modalities of the triple assessment of a breast lesion. Smears are examined for cellular atopy and cellular adhesion. Benign cells are regular in shape and size and tend to adhere to one another in clumps. Neoplastic cells vary in size, show nuclear pleomorphism or mitotic activity. Aspirates from cysts require cytological assessment only if bloodstained.

Answers

STATION 3.38

Assessment	Good	Adequate	Poor/not done
1 Appropriate introduction (full name and role)	☐	☐	☐
2 Informs patient of result	☐	☐	☐
3 Answers questions on the diagnosis with care	☐	☐	☐
4 Answers questions on outcome in broad, optimistic terms	☐	☐	☐
5 Ascertains if patient wishes to be involved in management decisions?	☐	☐	☐
6 Answers questions on treatment and side effects	☐	☐	☐
7 Does all the above in a fluent, empathetic and non-jargonistic manner	☐	☐	☐

Answers

Comment

If the patient already suspects the diagnosis, it should be confirmed gently. If the patient is unaware of the diagnosis, the results should be conveyed, giving time for the information to be understood. Occasionally, on being informed of the diagnosis, the patient may go into denial, when further discussion should be postponed to a meeting with the breast nurse counsellor (and if required, a clinical psychologist). Further, if the patient's partner does not wish her to be told of the diagnosis, this should be honoured as long as the patient does not actively seek information.

Should the patient not wish to be involved in management decisions, she must, nevertheless, be informed of the chosen protocol, its effectiveness and side-effects. If the patient is in denial of the diagnosis and rejects treatment, assistance from nurse counsellors, psychologist and the patient's family are required to bring her out of denial. Those patients who wish to participate in selecting treatment protocols must be given sufficient information and encouragement, as they will then be better prepared to tolerate the side-effects or to accept failures of treatment.

Chapter 4:
Ethics and Legal Medicine, including Consent and IV Procedures Answers

Chapter 4

Ethics and Legal Medicine, including Consent and IV Procedures Answers

STATION 4.1

Assessment	Good	Adequate	Poor/not done
1 Ascertains the time and size of the overdose	☐	☐	☐
2 Ascertains what the House Officer and A&E staff have already done (ie information given to patient)	☐	☐	☐
3 Establishes any clear reason(s)for the patient to refuse treatment	☐	☐	☐
4 Explains to the House Officer what can be done:	☐	☐	☐
If the patient is rational, one cannot force treatment on her	☐	☐	☐
Needs to explain clearly and simply the effects of the paracetamol overdose, (ie liver poisoning)	☐	☐	☐
Explain clearly and simply the treatment (ie intravenous Parvolex or oral N-acetyl cysteine)	☐	☐	☐
5 Checks that the House Officer has understood the process	☐	☐	☐

Comment

In this case the initial suicide attempt and the refusal of treatment in itself shows serious suicidal intent. The patient is placing her life at risk and may have an underlying depressive illness for which psychiatric care should be provided immediately. The implications of having or not having the treatment should be fully and clearly explained and the patient's understanding assessed.

The Court of Appeal has ruled that a patient lacks capacity only if impairment of the mind renders her or him unable to decide whether to consent or refuse treatment, and that if they lack capacity, seeking consent is futile. Treatment may be provided in these circumstances under the common law justification of necessity. The House of Lords has stated that a competent patient on reaching a balanced judgement on adequate information received may choose to reject medical advice for any or no reason. This patient's unequivocal assurance that her refusal is an informed decision should be documented. Such a patient may sue for battery and false imprisonment if treated against her will and when her refusal is respected there is no prospect of her (or her estate, if she dies) suing for negligence or negligent advice.

STATION 4.2a

Patient history

I am 56 years old and I have two daughters. I found out recently that the reason for my father's suicide was that he had just been diagnosed as having Huntington's chorea. I know very little about the disorder except that sufferers become demented and usually die prematurely. I understand that it is passed on through the genes, and this is why I asked for the test, which the other doctor organised. I do not want to tell my relatives, as I am frightened for myself and for their well-being. I could not face my daughters knowing that I might have given them a fatal illness, as I am sure they would never forgive me. I love my three brothers and two daughters, and would not want any harm to come to any of them. (When the doctor has clarified the situation sensitively), I will feel more reassured now and will agree to allow you to tell the rest of the family.

Assessment	Good	Adequate	Poor/not done
1 Appropriate introduction (full name and role)	☐	☐	☐
2 Establishes patient's understanding of Huntington's chorea	☐	☐	☐
3 Establishes patient's understanding about the inheritance/genetics of the disease	☐	☐	☐
4 Carefully elicits reasons why the patient does not want the family to know:			
Embarrassment – self/family	☐	☐	☐
Shame – self/family	☐	☐	☐
Protection – self/family	☐	☐	☐
Disclosure of father's/grandfather's illness	☐	☐	☐
Investigates family dynamics –possible conflicts between siblings/daughters and patient.	☐	☐	☐
Clarifies genetics and effects of disorder; patient's obligations	☐	☐	☐
Explains duties to patient –respect of patient's wishes, confidentiality	☐	☐	☐
Explains that he is obliged and able to inform the other family members without mentioning or involving the patient	☐	☐	☐
5 Non-judgemental and respectful of patient's feelings	☐	☐	☐

Answers

Comment

The BMA's code of practice on genetic counselling would argue that the patient's daughter, because she may be affected, is entitled to the information despite the patient's wishes. The Court of Appeal has held that information obtained in a confidential relationship may be disclosed if in the public interest. It would seem that a possibility of preventing the birth of a child with the disorder may be considered sufficient to merit disclosure. Further, the patient's daughter may, in the course of time, bring a case of negligence against you for failing in your duty to warn her of a foreseeable risk.

STATION 4.3a

Relative's history

I am the daughter of the patient, Mr Jones. My brother does not really know what is going on and is unable to attend. I am the patient's primary carer. In the last few months I have had to do all his cleaning, washing, bathing and shopping. My father has become increasingly confused and is incontinent of urine all the time. He is often found on the floor, and in the last few weeks has been wandering outside. He leaves the gas on and often mistakes the oven for the fridge. (Maggots were found in the oven.) I can't cope with him any more and don't see why everyone else is trying to let him go home, where he is plainly unsafe. My daughter has been ill over the last week, so I have been unable to come to the hospital and see my father.

Assessment	Good	Adequate	Poor/not done
1 Appropriate introduction (full name and role)	☐	☐	☐
2 Establishes ground rules of the meeting: chairperson, time limits of the meeting, when questions should be asked	☐	☐	☐
3 Establishes reasons for the meeting	☐	☐	☐
4 Establishes patient's case from the medical notes	☐	☐	☐
5 Presents other healthcare members' reports/invites them to report	☐	☐	☐
6 Invites relatives to air their concerns	☐	☐	☐
7 Addresses patient's concerns in a logical manner (eg gas being capped off, cognitive function much improved)	☐	☐	☐
8 Invites patient to air his views	☐	☐	☐
9 Ensures that patient is respected	☐	☐	☐
10 Agrees/establishes compromise situation	☐	☐	☐
11 Summarises action plan	☐	☐	☐
12 Ensures all parties are in agreement and understand the situation	☐	☐	☐
13 Takes organised, systematic approach	☐	☐	☐

Comment

This situation has arisen because of an organic illness. The urinary-tract infection has caused the insidious worsening of his general state and has led the daughter to feel that her father is no longer coping, and has become too difficult for her to manage. Through medical treatment and good rehabilitation, the patient is now much improved. Simple communication between the relatives and staff, and demonstration of the 'new, improved' Mr Jones, would probably have obviated the need for the care-planning meeting. In such cases the staff must assess the patient when at his/her best. Therapies must have been allowed to take effect before a home visit or ward assessment. If the patient is considered of 'reasonable cognitive ability', every avenue must be explored to allow him or her to go home. All safety precautions must be implemented, the patient fully briefed and a 'trial of failure' initiated: where everyone, but the patient, is convinced he/she will probably fail at home. Through maximising home support and helping relatives cope, this trial of failure is often successful for relatively lengthy periods.

STATION 4.4a

Comment

This situation encompasses a very important principle, that of appropriateness of care. Although increasing age is often quoted as a negative prognostic factor, it is usually the only factor considered in such situations. In this situation the patient with the worst prognosis is, in fact, the young 24-year-old man. The appropriateness of treating a man with acquired immune deficiency syndrome (AIDS) and multi-organ failure is not the question, but the appropriateness of treating him at the expense of one of the other patients is. If the consultant in charge of the AIDS patient's case decides that his ventilation should be continued, this patient should not be moved, as he is most unwell and the least likely to survive transfer. The 83-year-old man is also unlikely to survive a prolonged transfer, so it is one of the other patients who should be moved to another hospital.

Answers

STATION 4.5

Patient history

I am a 30-year-old university graduate and couldn't get any job at all until 6 months ago. I have been driving a minicab for a local firm and have been earning good money. Although I know it is totally illegal, I haven't informed the driver and vehicle licensing centre (DVLC) or my employer that I am epileptic. I was diagnosed as having epilepsy 5 years ago, and haven't had a seizure for the last 10 months. This must mean that I am cured! I understand that I should be able to drive again but not for another year or so. I can't give up my job, as my wife is expecting our second child in 3 months.

Assessment	Good	Adequate	Poor/not done
1 Appropriate introduction (full name and role)	☐	☐	☐
2 Establishes why the patient is attending	☐	☐	☐
3 Establishes the patient's control of seizures and adherence to treatment	☐	☐	☐
4 Establishes patient's understanding of the law regarding epilepsy and driving	☐	☐	☐
5 Establishes the reasons why the patient continues to drive	☐	☐	☐
6 Looks for possible areas of compromise (eg 6 weeks' sick leave/holidays;	☐	☐	☐
explanation to employer with GP support; social services support)	☐	☐	☐
7 Raises issues of family and social obligations	☐	☐	☐
8 Informs the patient of the legal obligation for the doctor to inform the DVLC	☐	☐	☐
9 Agrees on a compromise with the patient and reiterates plan	☐	☐	☐
SP to mark			
10 The doctor listened to and acknowledged my concerns	☐	☐	☐
11 I felt supported by this doctor	☐	☐	☐

Answers

Comment

The BMA code of practice states that when there is a conflict between a doctor's duty to society and patient confidentiality, the doctor should seek to persuade the patient to disclose the information, or to give permission for the doctor to disclose it. The prevention of potential harm to society should supersede the duty of confidentiality. In this case the patient is wrong. The law states that a patient must be fit-free for one year, or have had only nocturnal seizures for 3 or more years to be able to drive. Since the patient has been fit-free for 10 months, he could negotiate with his employer, with the GP's help, to keep his job. In 2 months, if still fit-free, he would be able to drive again legally.

Answers

STATION 4.6a

Patient history

I am a 52-year-old schoolteacher. My husband died in a road traffic accident 5 years ago, and I have been drowning my sorrows ever since. My GP performed some routine blood tests on me about 3 months ago, and I was sent to see the liver specialist and told to cut down on my drinking. I am a little nervous but otherwise have no problems with the biopsy. The consultant told me it was a small cut on the right side of my tummy to get a small piece of liver.

Assessment	Good	Adequate	Poor/not done
1 Appropriate introduction (full name and role)	☐	☐	☐
2 Explains what interview will be about	☐	☐	☐
3 Establishes patient identity and reason for admission	☐	☐	☐
4 Establishes patient's present understanding of the procedure	☐	☐	☐
5 Explains procedure:			
Patient to lie flat on the bed *Duration of the procedure*	☐	☐	☐
Patient able to hold a deep breath for 10 seconds	☐	☐	☐
Procedure performed under local anaesthetic	☐	☐	☐
Skin cleaned and infiltrated with local anaesthetic	☐	☐	☐
Small incision made over lateral aspect of the right upper quadrant	☐	☐	☐
Needle passed into the liver and a small amount removed	☐	☐	☐
6 Common side-effects explained	☐	☐	☐
7 Uncommon side-effects explained	☐	☐	☐
8 Post-procedure period explained	☐	☐	☐

Answers

9 'Chunks' information to help retention   ☐   ☐   ☐

10 Invites patient questions, and answers
    appropriately   ☐   ☐   ☐

11 Gives clear, jargon-free explanation.   ☐   ☐   ☐

12 Checks patient's understanding of
    information   ☐   ☐   ☐

13 When asked, states that the procedure
    cannot be performed until FBC and INR
    are known   ☐   ☐   ☐

14 Asks patient to sign consent form   ☐   ☐   ☐

15 Systematic, organised approach   ☐   ☐   ☐

Comment

Contraindications to this procedure include:

(a) Patient unable to lie flat or take deep breath

(b) Local infection of skin

(c) Ascites

(d) Intra-abdominal sepsis

(e) Deranged clotting (INR >1.4)

(f) Platelets <80+000

Answers

STATION 4.7a

Patient history

I am 43 years old and have received a letter from the hospital asking me to attend today for endoscopy. No one has explained anything to me, and I have no idea what this is all about. I would like the situation clearly explained. My doctor did mention that I am anaemic and that this may need looking into. He said something about a special test but nothing else. I feel quite cross that no one bothered to give me any information.

Assessment	Good	Adequate	Poor/not done
1 Appropriate introduction (full name and role)	☐	☐	☐
2 Explains purpose of interview	☐	☐	☐
3 Establishes patient identity and reason for procedure	☐	☐	☐
4 Explains the following elements of the procedure:			
Performed normally with local anaesthetic spray	☐	☐	☐
Can be given sedation but not a general anaesthetic	☐	☐	☐
Endoscope (telescope/instrument) is about 1 cm in diameter passed down into stomach	☐	☐	☐
Look down into oesophagus (gullet), stomach and first part of bowel	☐	☐	☐
Can take small pieces of the lining (biopsies) to look at under microscope	☐	☐	☐
Uncomfortable but no pain during procedure	☐	☐	☐
Mentions common side-effects – sore throat and gullet	☐	☐	☐
Mentions rare side-effects – Oesophageal tear	☐	☐	☐

Mediastinitis	☐	☐	☐
Pneumomediastinum	☐	☐	☐
5 'Chunks' information to help retention	☐	☐	☐
6 Gives clear, jargon-free explanation	☐	☐	☐
7 Invites patient questions, and answers appropriately	☐	☐	☐
8 Checks patient's understanding of information	☐	☐	☐
9 Systematic, organised approach	☐	☐	☐

SP to mark:

10 The doctor listened to my concerns	☐	☐	☐

Comment

Indications for upper GI endoscopy:

Acute: Upper GI bleed/haematemesis or melaena

Acute oesophageal obstruction.

Chronic: Investigation of dysphagia, hypochromic microcytic anaemia, weight loss, vomiting, dyspepsia, celiac disease/malabsorption.

Answers

STATION 4.8a

Patient history

I am 62 years old and a retired school teacher. I am being investigated for constipation and weight loss. I am very concerned that I may have cancer of the bowel, because this is what my sister died of. She had a miserable and painful death. My GP described the colonoscopy to me briefly and said the doctors would pass a camera into my bowel. I am not sure what this means.

Assessment	Good	Adequate	Poor/not done
1 Appropriate introduction (name and role)	☐	☐	☐
2 Explains purpose of interview	☐	☐	☐
3 Establishes patient identity and reason for attendance	☐	☐	☐
4 Establishes patient's present understanding of the procedure.	☐	☐	☐
5 Explains the elements of the procedure:			
Procedure performed using intravenous sedation	☐	☐	☐
Endoscope passed in through anus up into the bowel	☐	☐	☐
Endoscope is about 1 cm in diameter, flexible, and carries a fibre-optic light allowing the operator to see inside the bowel	☐	☐	☐
Allows biopsies to be taken	☐	☐	☐
6 Mentions common side-effects – PR bleeding; discomfort during procedure	☐	☐	☐
7 Mentions uncommon side-effects – small tears of bowel treated conservatively; larger tears of bowel requiring operation	☐	☐	☐
8 Gives clear, jargon-free explanation	☐	☐	☐

Answers

9 'Chunks' information to help retention ☐ ☐ ☐

10 Invites patient questions and addresses anxieties ☐ ☐ ☐

11 Checks patient's understanding of information ☐ ☐ ☐

12 Systematic, organised approach ☐ ☐ ☐

SP to mark

13 This doctor was empathic ☐ ☐ ☐

Comment

Indications for colonoscopy:

Acute: Bleeding from the lower bowel.

Chronic: Investigation of weight loss, change in bowel habit, bleeding or mucus PR, hypochromic microcytic anaemia.

STATION 4.9a

Patient history

I am 36 years old and work in a factory. I have been getting pain in the top right part of my tummy for the last 6–8 months. The pain is particularly bad after fried foods. The pain was so bad 3 days ago that I called out my GP and I was admitted to hospital. Yesterday I had a scan, which showed that a gallstone was blocking up my liver. I have been told that I need a special test which allows the doctors to look inside my bowel, near the liver, and remove the stone. I am happy to have this procedure, but I do not understand how all organs are 'joined' together, or how they will manage to get the gallstone out without opening me up.

Assessment	Good	Adequate	Poor/not done
1 Appropriate introduction (full name and role)	☐	☐	☐
2 Establishes the patient's identity and reason for the ERCP	☐	☐	☐
3 Establishes patient's present understanding of endoscopic retrograde cholangiopancreatography (ERCP)	☐	☐	☐
4 Gives clear, jargon-free explanation	☐	☐	☐
5 Explains the following elements of the procedure:			
Procedure is performed under intravenous sedation, not general anaesthetic	☐	☐	☐
Endoscope is about 1 cm in diameter. It is flexible and carries a fibre-optic light which allows the operator to see inside the bowel	☐	☐	☐
Endoscope is passed down through the gullet into the first part of the bowel The sphincter of Oddi is identified and cut, using instrument passed down the endoscope	☐	☐	☐
Metal cage/basket is passed up into the biliary tree	☐	☐	☐

Answers

Gallstone is removed using the cage
If the procedure is unsuccessful,further
attempts may be undertaken   ☐   ☐   ☐

Patient may require surgical
Intervention   ☐   ☐   ☐

6 Offers to draw or show diagram to clarify
   anatomy   ☐   ☐   ☐

7 Invites patient questions, and answers
   appropriately   ☐   ☐   ☐

8 Checks patient's understanding of
   information   ☐   ☐   ☐

9 Systematic, organised approach   ☐   ☐   ☐

SP to mark

10 I understand the explanation   ☐   ☐   ☐

Comment

The use of ERCP is quite specific. Most patients having an ERCP will also have to give consent for the use of contrast media being injected through the sphincter of Oddi and X-ray images being taken of the resulting patterns through the biliary tree and pancreatic ducts. Consent must be obtained for sphincterotomy which frequently accompanies ERCP. One specific use of ERCP is the insertion of stents to unplug biliary ducts in benign and malignant conditions. All patients for ERCP receive prophylactic anitbiotics for 24 hours pre- and post-procedure, and should be fasting for 8 hours pre-procedure. It is often difficult for patients to conceptualise the anatomy and how stents/wire baskets may be sited using an endoscope. ERCP is often best explained using a diagram.

Answers

STATION 4.10a

Patient history

I am 43 years old and was admitted to hospital 2 days ago with a fever, exertional dyspnoea and lethargy. I have been told I have a new heart murmur and it is suspected I have an infection on the heart valve. I know this procedure is to look at the heart valves and to try to see if they are damaged, but I have not been told anything else. I am a little anxious about the whole thing and wondered if it is possible to be put to sleep for the procedure.

Assessment	Good	Adequate	Poor/not done
1 Appropriate introduction (full name and role)	☐	☐	☐
2 Explains purpose of interview	☐	☐	☐
3 Establishes present understanding of the procedure	☐	☐	☐
4 Explains the procedure:			
Procedure performed with patient conscious	☐	☐	☐
Patients can be given injection to make them sleepy	☐	☐	☐
Instrument is about 3-4 cm at its thickest	☐	☐	☐
The procedure should be no more than uncomfortable	☐	☐	☐
5 Mentions the common complications – sore throat and oesophagus	☐	☐	☐
6 Mentions the uncommon complications – oesophagus rupture; mediastinal sepsis; death	☐	☐	☐
7 Re-establishes patient understanding of procedure	☐	☐	☐
8 'Chunks' information to help retention	☐	☐	☐
9 Gives clear, jargon-free explanation	☐	☐	☐

Answers

10 Invites questions and answers
    appropriately   ☐   ☐   ☐

11 Checks patient's understanding of
    information   ☐   ☐   ☐

12 Systematic, organised approach   ☐   ☐   ☐

SP to mark:

13 The doctor was empathic   ☐   ☐   ☐

Comment

Transoesophageal echocardiogram requires the placement of the echo probe in the gullet adjacent to the heart and moved to obtain adequate ciné imaging of valvular anatomy and function.

Answers

STATION 4.11a

Patient history

I am 53 years old and am a headmaster. I had a 'heart attack' 6 months ago. I saw the consultant cardiologist 2 weeks ago, who thought I should have a 'catheter' test to see how bad the damage is to the blood vessels supplying the heart. I have not been told very much but would like to know as much as possible. I am otherwise well and can lie flat in bed with no problems. I have never had any reactions to any medications.

(NB. Ask the doctor specifically about any concerns you may have.)

Assessment	Good	Adequate	Poor/not done
1 Appropriate introduction (full name and role) and establishes patient's identity	☐	☐	☐
2 Explains purpose of interview	☐	☐	☐
3 Establishes present understanding of the procedure	☐	☐	☐
4 Explains the elements of the procedure:			
Performed under local anaesthetic	☐	☐	☐
Injection into the groin through which a thin tube is placed	☐	☐	☐
Contrast medium is injected through the tube/cine film is taken	☐	☐	☐
5 Explains common complications – reaction to contrast medium and bruising in the groin	☐	☐	☐
6 Explains the uncommon complications – femoral false aneurysm and rupture of coronary vessel	☐	☐	☐
7 Specifically explains the risk and benefits of the procedure – including mortality	☐	☐	☐
8 'Chunks' information to help retention	☐	☐	☐
9 Gives clear, jargon-free explanation	☐	☐	☐

10 Invites patient questions and deals with
    them in an appropriate manner   ☐   ☐   ☐

11 Establishes the patient understanding at
    the end of the explanation   ☐   ☐   ☐

12 Asks patient whether he wishes to sign
    consent form   ☐   ☐   ☐

13 Systematic, organised approach   ☐   ☐   ☐

Answers

STATION 4.12

Assessment	Good	Adequate	Poor/not done
1 Appropriate introduction (full name and role)	☐	☐	☐
2 Establishes and checks the patient's identity	☐	☐	☐
3 Explains the procedure to the patient in a clear manner	☐	☐	☐
4 Checks that the correct equipment is available: needle/vacutainer or syringe, alcohol wipe, FBC bottle, tourniquet, gloves	☐	☐	☐
5 Performs the procedure in the following steps:			
Puts on gloves		☐	☐
Places tourniquet on the arm correctly		☐	☐
Selects appropriate vein to site cannula		☐	☐
Cleans skin with alcohol wipe		☐	☐
Connects needle/vacutainer or syringe correctly		☐	☐
Warns patient of 'sharp scratch'		☐	☐
Inserts needle at approximately 35–45°		☐	☐
Withdraws appropriate amount of blood (FBC 1–4 ml)		☐	☐
Releases tourniquet		☐	☐
Withdraws the needle		☐	☐
Covers puncture site with cotton wool or alcohol wipe, asking the patient to press on the area		☐	☐
Does all in as clean a manner as possible		☐	☐
Disposes of sharps appropriately		☐	☐
States would label the bottle correctly and fill in appropriate FBC form	☐	☐	☐
6 Does all in a fluent, professional manner	☐	☐	☐

Answers

STATION 4.13

Assessment	Good	Adequate	Poor/not done
1 Appropriate introduction (full name and role)	☐	☐	☐
2 Establishes identity of the patient	☐	☐	☐
3 Explains the procedure to the patient in a clear manner	☐	☐	☐
4 Checks the right equipment is present (ie intravenous cannula, alcohol wipe, tourniquet, vecafix or similar dressing for cannula,normal saline flush, gloves)	☐	☐	☐
5 Candidate washes their hands using the alcohol handwash provided (no marks if candidate only expresses the need to wash if handwash is provided)	☐	☐	☐
6 Performs the procedure in the following steps:			
Puts on gloves		☐	☐
Places the tourniquet on the arm correctly		☐	☐
Selects appropriate vein to site cannula		☐	☐
Cleans skin with alcohol wipe		☐	☐
Warns patient of 'sharp scratch'		☐	☐
Passes cannula through skin at 35–45°		☐	☐
Looks/obtains flashback into cannula chamber		☐	☐
Releases tourniquet		☐	☐
Inserts cannula while withdrawing introducer		☐	☐
Pushes on tip of cannula, or asks patient to elevate arm (to stop bleeding as introducer is withdrawn)		☐	☐
Replaces cap over end of cannula		☐	☐
Secures cannula with dressing		☐	☐

Answers

	Good	Adequate	Poor/not done
Flushes cannula using saline flush		☐	☐
Does all in as clean a manner as possible		☐	☐
Disposes of sharps appropriately		☐	☐
7 Does all in a fluent, professional manner	☐	☐	☐

STATION 4.14

Assessment	Good	Adequate	Poor/not done
1 Appropriate introduction (full name and role); establishes the patient's identity	☐	☐	☐
2 Explains procedure to the patient in a clear manner	☐	☐	☐
3 Checks fluid prescription on chart, patient's details and fluid provided	☐	☐	☐
4 Checks that all correct equipment is present (eg normal saline + 20 mmol KCl, giving set and drip stand or equivalent)	☐	☐	☐
5 Candidate washes their hands using the alcohol handwash provided (no marks if candidate only expresses the need to wash if handwash is provided)	☐	☐	☐
6 Puts on gloves		☐	☐
7 Connects giving set to intravenous fluid correctly	☐	☐	☐
8 Runs through fluid so giving set is appropriately filled, removing air bubbles	☐	☐	☐
9 Removes cannula cap and attaches fluid correctly	☐	☐	☐
10 Ensures fluid is running easily into vein without causing pain/burning sensation.	☐	☐	☐
11 Ensures giving set is securely attached to the patient and cannula (may use a bandage)	☐	☐	☐
11 Does all in a fluent, professional manner	☐	☐	☐

STATION 4.15

Assessment	Good	Adequate	Poor/not done
1 Appropriate introduction (full name and role)	☐	☐	☐
2 Establishes patient identity	☐	☐	☐
3 Explains procedure to patient in a clear manner	☐	☐	☐
4 Checks that the correct equipment is rresent (ie saline flush, needles, syringes, antibiotic, mixing fluid)	☐	☐	
5 Checks the prescription chart, antibiotic and dose against patient identity bracelet	☐	☐	☐
6 Checks the patient has no known drug allergy	☐	☐	☐
7 Candidate washes their hands using the alcohol handwash provided (no marks if candidate only expresses the need to wash if handwash is provided)	☐	☐	☐
8 Performs the procedure as follows: *Puts gloves on*		☐	☐
Removes seal on antibiotic vial *Cleans top of antibiotic vial with alcohol wipe*		☐	☐
Draws up mixing fluid (eg water for injection)		☐	☐
Injects mixing fluid into antibiotic vial		☐	☐
Mixes antibiotic/fluid appropriately		☐	☐
Draws back antibiotic		☐	☐
Cleans cannula portal with alcohol wipe		☐	☐
Injects antibiotic slowly		☐	☐
Flushes cannula with saline flush		☐	☐
Closes cannula portal		☐	☐

Answers

Disposes of sharps and other materials
appropriately ☐ ☐

9 Does all in a fluent, professional manner ☐ ☐ ☐

Mock Exam

The table contains seven examinations of 16 stations taken from the text, each lasts two hours – this allows three five minute rest stations in examination 2 and two rest stations in the other examinations at convenient times. The symbol + indicates a 10, rather than the usual 5, minute station, and ++ an extra 5 minute preparation for a 10 minute station. A 'subject' is needed to give the history, where this is provided in the text answer, and also for examination stations when stated.

Station	1	2	3	4	5	6	7
1	1.1	1.2	1.3	1.4+	1.5	1.6	1.7
2	1.8+	1.9	1.10	1.17	1.11+	1.12++	1.14++
3	1.13++	1.5++	1.16	1.18	1.19	1.20	1.22+
4	1.21+	1.25+	1.24+	1.25+	1.26	1.27	1.28
5	1.29	2.1	2.2	2.3	2.4+	2.5+	2.6
6	2.7	2.5	2.9	2.10	2.13	2.15	2.11
7	2.14+	2.12+	2.16	2.17	2.18	2.19	2.20
8	2.21	2.22	2.23	2.24	2.25	2.26	2.27
9	2.28	2.29+	2.30+	2.31	2.33+	3.1+	3.3
10	3.4	3.5	3.6	3.7+	3.10	3.9	3.8
11	3.11	3.12	3.13+	3.14	3.15	3.18	3.17
12	3.16	3.20	3.21	3.19	3.22	3.23	3.24
13	3.25	3.27	3.26	3.34	3.28	3.29+	3.30+
14	3.31	3.32	3.33	3.38	3.35	3.36	3.37
15	4.10+	4.5+	4.3++	4.4++	4.16++	4.7+	4.1+
16	4.12	4.11+	4.13	4.8+	4.14	4.15	4.9+

The OSCE marking scheme

Traditionally, academic assessment has been 'norm' referenced, whereby candidates are compared to one another and are ranked from the best to the worst. In recent years the value of 'norm' referencing has come under question and 'criterion' referencing has become more accepted.

Criterion-referenced assessment is not new, the most obvious examples being the driving test and swimming life saving assessments. In both these examples a candidate must demonstrate a 'minimum competency level' for the given skills, ie driving a motor vehicle or saving a drowning person. Unlike traditional, norm-referenced assessment, there is no division of candidates into excellent, good, average, unsatisfactory and poor; there is only pass (competent) and fail (not competent).

Criterion referencing is easily applied to the OSCE format. A committee of examiners meets several months prior to the examinations and, through discussion, sets a minimum competency score, ie a passing score, for each given station. This score reflects what a candidate taking the OSCE should be reasonably expected to achieve, given their expected core knowledge, the time restrictions and the stress of the examination. These, in turn, should be reflected in the validity of the OSCE.

In volumes 1 and 2 the checklists are divided into three columns headed **Good**, **Adequate** and **Poor/not done**. These headings subdivide students into good, average and poor, where poor candidates do not demonstrate an acceptable level of competence, i.e. fail. However, in many medical establishments, the division of good and average candidates is regarded as old fashioned, regressing back to norm referencing and therefore the headings may read **Adequate or competent**, **Attempted but unsatisfactory** and **Not done**.

Some medical colleges apply weighting of individual items within a checklist. For instance, the initial item on each checklist 'Appropriate introduction (full name and role)', may have a maximum score of two marks if performed well, whereas another item, eg auscultating the four areas of the heart correctly, may carry 5 marks if performed well. Both would be given a lesser mark if performed adequately and 0 marks if not done at all. We have chosen not to weight individual items in our checklists. This is because:

(i)   We feel that weighting of items in this way does not improve the discriminatory power of the examination.

(ii)   We think students should be discerning enough to realise which are the important key points that will be more heavily weighted in a checklist.

We have, therefore, generally used 3 columns for our checklists, **Good**, **Adequate** and **Poor/not done**, carrying 3, 2 and 0 marks respectively. Certain checklists, however, only have 2 columns, i.e. Adequate and Not done. These are typically items which are required to be named, e.g. risk factors for a DVT or contraindications to a given treatment. One can only mention them or not and for this reason a 'good column' is not applicable. In such cases 1 mark is given for adequate column and zero for the Poor/not done column.

To obtain the total score

For each station, minimum competency or pass mark is calculated by a committee of examiners/experts. If a candidate scores each item as 'adequate' this will equate to the 'pass' mark. A candidate should therefore aim to get an adequate or good for each item. If one scores adequate or poor/not done in the majority of items, this implies a lack of knowledge or areas of weakness and should be used to direct the student's learning.

In most OSCEs the stations are deemed to be as important as one another, so that the mean pass mark of the total number of stations is taken as the pass mark for the overall examination. If individual stations are important in terms of 'must pass', a weighting system may be applied to calculate the overall pass mark.

We have used one other style of marking whereby the station poses a series of questions to the student regarding an investigation, e.g. an abdominal radiograph, or a given scenario, e.g. management of a head injury patient. Examiners may consider that such answers should also carry serious consequences for the candidate, such as an outright failure on that question.

Establishing rapport with a patient is essential in a doctor-patient relationship. At the initial meeting, greetings and introductions help to put the patient at ease and ensure patient co-operation with the history and/or examination. In these stations, therefore, marks are allocated for such interaction. Positive criteria include empathy, putting a patient at their ease and establishing their confidence by careful listening and responding to verbal and non-verbal cues.

Revision Checklist

Paediatrics

Neonatology

Respiratory distress syndrome ☐
Prematurity ☐
Birth asphyxia ☐
Neonatal jaundice ☐
Intrauterine growth retardation ☐
Congenital heart disease ☐
Talipes ☐
Hypoglycaemia ☐
Dysmorphic Syndromes ☐
Congenital dislocation of the hips ☐
Cleft lip and palate ☐
Congenital infections ☐
Neural tube defects ☐

Respiratory and Airway

Asthma ☐
Cystic fibrosis ☐
Bronchiolitis ☐
Pneumonia ☐
Epiglottitis ☐
Croup (Laryngotracheobronchitis) ☐
Otitis media ☐
Tonsillitis ☐

Heart and Cardiovascular

VSD ☐
Fallot's tetralogy ☐
Innocent murmurs ☐
Cyanotic heart defects ☐
Other acyanotic heart defects ☐
Coarctation of aorta ☐

Neurology and Development

Febrile fits ☐
Cerebral palsy ☐
Types of fits ☐
Down's syndrome ☐

Developmental delay ☐

Muscular dystrophy ☐

Children with special needs ☐

Language delay ☐

Migraine ☐

Squint ☐

Autism

Urinary Tract and Nephrology

Urinary Tract Infection ☐

Nephrotic syndrome ☐

Undescended testes ☐

Chronic renal failure ☐

Acute renal failure ☐

Gastro-Intestinal Disease

Coeliac disease ☐

Gastro-oesophageal reflux ☐

The acute abdomen in children ☐

Hernias ☐

Intussusception ☐

Hirschsprung's disease ☐

Pyloric stenosis ☐

Inflammatory bowel diseases ☐

Metabolic and Endocrine

Diabetes mellitus ☐

Failure to thrive ☐

Hypothyroidism ☐

Puberty ☐

Growth hormone Deficiency ☐

Congenital adrenal Hyperplasia ☐

Phenylketonuria ☐

Inborn errors of metabolism ☐

Immunology, Allergy, Dermatology

Eczema ☐

Nappy rash ☐

Substance allergies ☐

Henoch–Schonlein purpura ☐

Birth marks ☐

Neonatal skin disorders ☐

Immunodeficiencies ☐

Infections

Gastroenteritis ☐

Meningitis ☐

Meningococcal septicaemia ☐

AIDS

Staphylococcal Infections ☐

Streptococcal Infections ☐

Chicken pox ☐

Pertussis ☐

Measles/Mumps/Rubella ☐

Malaria ☐

TB ☐

Hepatitis ☐

EBV and CMV ☐

Child Psychiatry and Aspects of Social medicine

Sudden infant death ☐

Enuresis ☐

Child abuse ☐

Reaction to chronic disease ☐

Encopresis ☐

School refusal ☐

Hyperactivity ☐

Munchausen by Proxy ☐

Autism ☐

Sleep problems ☐

Parasuicide and Suicide ☐

Musculoskeletal and Joint

Septic arthritis ☐

Juvenile rheumatoid arthritis (JCA) ☐

Rickets ☐

Haematology

Iron deficiency anaemia ☐

Sickle cell disease in children ☐

Haemoglobinopathies in children ☐

Idiopathic thrombocytopaenia ☐

Overview of the management of malignancy in children ☐

Acute Lymphoblastic leukaemia ☐

Wilm's tumour ☐

Neuroblastoma ☐

Obstetrics, Newborn and Gynaecology

Antenatal care ☐
Hypertension and diabetes in pregnancy ☐
Ante- and post- partum haemorrhage ☐
Eclampsia ☐
Assessment of newborn ☐
Foetal distress ☐
Infertility ☐
Ectopic pregnancy ☐
Hydatidform mole ☐
Endometriosis ☐
Fibroids and uterine cancer ☐
Cervical erosions and cancer ☐

Endocrinology and Breast

Diabetes mellitus ☐
Diabetes insipidus ☐
Toxic and non-toxic goitre ☐
Parathyroid disease ☐
Acromegaly ☐
Addison's disease ☐
Conn's syndrome ☐
Cushing's disease ☐
Breast Cancer ☐
Urothelial tumours ☐
Prostatism and urinary retention ☐
Urinary infections ☐
Testicular descent and tumours ☐

Ethics and Legal Medicine

Patient's right to know ☐
Patient confidentiality ☐
Informed consent ☐
Sectioning psychiatric patients ☐
Organ donation ☐
In-vitro fertilisation ☐
Terminal care ☐

Recommended Reading list

Medical Texts

Hutchinson's Clinical Methods: Hutchinson R and Swash M, 21st edition, W B Saunders 2001.

Davidson's Principles and Practice of Medicine: Edwards CRW, Bouchier IAD, Haslett C and Chilvers ER (editors), 19th edition, Churchill Livingstone 2002.

Clinical Medicine: Kumar P and Clark M (editors), 5th edition, Saunders 2002.

Lecture Notes on Dermatology: Graham-Brown RAC, Burns T, 8th edition, Blackwell Science 2002.

Examining Patients: An Introduction to Clinical Medicine: Toghill PJ (editor), 2nd edition, Edward Arnold 1994.

Lecture Notes on Clinical Medicine: Rubenstein D, Bradley JR and Wayne D, 6th edition, Blackwell Science 2002.

Surgical Texts

Hamilton Bailey's Demonstrations of Physical Signs in Clinical Surgery: Lumley JSP, 18th edition, Butterworth Heinemann 1997.

Lecture Notes on General Surgery: Watson JE, Ellis H and Calne R, 10th edition, Blackwell Science 2002.

The Washington Manual of Surgery: Doherty GM (editor), 2nd edition, Lippincott, Williams and Wilkins 1999.

Bailey and Love's Short Practice of Surgery: Russell RCG, Williams NS, Bulstrode CJK (editors), 24th edition, Hodder Arnold 2004.

Obstetrics and Gynaecology Texts

ABC of Antenatal Care: Chamberlain G, Morgan M, 4th edition, BMJ 2002.

Lecture Notes in Obstetrics and Gynaecology: Hamilton-Fairley D, 2nd edition, Blackwell Science 2004.

Index

*Page numbers in normal text refer to the questions, page numbers in **bold** refer to the answers.*